MANAGING PAIN BEFORE IT MANAGES YOU

Health Education Department & Library
3285 Claremont Way
Napa, CA. 94558

Open: Monday – Thursday 9:00 a.m. - 5:00 p.m.
(closed for lunch 12:30 p.m. - 1:30 p.m.)

707-258-4490

Late Fee Policy
Late fees are accrued at <u>$.25 cents per day</u> for each item past the return due date.

You must call to extend your due date **before** the item is overdue. (max 1 week extension)

> OVERDUE ITEMS CANNOT BE EXTENDED.

The Outside Book Drop Box
(available 24 hours a day) is located in front of the Claremont Building (by the patient drop off area)

Managing Pain Before It Manages You

Revised Edition

MARGARET A. CAUDILL, MD, PhD

Foreword by Herbert Benson, MD

THE GUILFORD PRESS
New York / London

© 2002 The Guilford Press
A Division of Guilford Publications, Inc.
72 Spring Street, New York, NY 10012
www.guilford.com

Printed in the United States of America

This book is printed on acid-free paper.

Last digit is print number: 9 8 7 6 5 4 3 2 1

Library of Congress Cataloging-in-Publication Data

Caudill, Margaret.
    Managing pain before it manages you / Margaret A. Caudill; foreword
by Herbert Benson.—Rev. ed.
        p.   cm.
    Includes bibliographical references and index.
    ISBN 1-57230-718-8 (pbk.)
    1. Pain—Popular works. I. Title.
RB127 .C384 2002
616′.0472—dc21

                                                                2001040959

Names and identifying details of all patients' stories have been changed to
protect their anonymity. They are composites of true patient stories.

The following publishers have generously given permission to use extended
quotations from copyrighted works: The Octagon Press (London) for excerpts
from *The Pleasantries of the Incredible Mulla Nasrudin* and *The Subtleties of the
Inimitable Mulla Nasrudin and The Exploits of the Incomparable Mulla Nasrudin*
by Idries Shah (copyright 1983 by Octagon Press, Ltd.); Beyond Words
Publishing (Hillsboro, OR), for an excerpt from *There's a Hole in My Sidewalk* by
Portia Nelson (copyright 1993 by Beyond Words Publishing).

To the patients who have instructed me in the tenacity
of the human spirit

To my family—Richard, Laura, and Paul

Contents

Foreword

Dr. Margaret Caudill has been my pain doctor as well as a professional colleague for many years. From relatively simple joint problems to severe injuries from an accident, she provided me with wise and successful pain management. I am deeply grateful and proud to be an associate of hers.

Dr. Caudill's expertise in pain reflects her extensive experience in wedding mind–body approaches with pain medications, therapeutic exercises, and diet. She has developed a clinically tested program recognized throughout the world. Her program for chronic pain had been scientifically proven to significantly lessen anxiety and depression, as well as anger and hostility. It diminishes the interference in life that comes with chronic pain; there is less overall distress; and in many cases the severity of pain is reduced. These improvements very frequently occur along with decreased use of pain medications, and so successful is her approach that patients on average reduce their visits to physicians by 36% for years following treatments.

Dr. Caudill has achieved these remarkable results by coupling what people can do for themselves along with state-of-the-art medical treatments. The program is in use at the Beth Israel Deaconess Medical Center in Boston, at the Dartmouth Hitchcock Clinic in Manchester, New Hampshire, and at Mind/Body Medical Institute affiliates around the country. *Managing Pain Before It Manages You* is the book used by patients and health professionals in these clinics.

The publication of *Managing Pain Before It Manages You* allows those of you who are not participating in a formally structured program to make use of its approach. You may also use it along with a pain regimen prescribed by your health care provider. Or you may find that your health care provider has prescribed it for you. The book is user-friendly, providing practical advice in an engaging fashion.

Those who have used this approach report that in addition to lessening their suffering from pain, they have learned how to apply its principles to other aspects of their lives. They communicate better, have a more positive attitude, and frequently achieve other elusive health goals. Overall, they report having gained more control over their lives.

Managing Pain Before It Manages You reflects the author's caring and compassion, as well as her experience and wisdom. Successful mind–body approaches require these qualities. Many patients erroneously believe that mind–body treatments mean their pain is "only in their heads." This is not what Dr. Caudill teaches. Rather, she expertly guides you through these considerations by teaching beneficial aspects of mind–body interactions to help you in improving your entire life.

I trust that your use of the approach in *Managing Pain Before It Manages You* will aid you as much as it has the many thousands who have already benefited from it.

Herbert Benson, MD
Harvard Medical School
Beth Israel Deaconess Medical Center

Acknowledgments

It is important to acknowledge the very real and crucial contributions of my colleagues Richard Schnable, Margaret Ennis, Carol Wells-Federman, and Paul Arnstein. Over the years, our dialogues and cumulative experience have created the Chronic Pain Management Program. It is impossible to distinguish where their ideas end and mine begin.

I would also like to acknowledge the invaluable support of my colleagues at the Division of Behavioral Medicine, the Mind/Body Medical Institute, and the Arnold Pain Center at the Beth Israel Deaconess Medical Center in Boston, Massachusetts, as well as those at the Dartmouth Hitchcock Clinic in New Hampshire. A special thanks to Nancy L. Josephson, who is responsible for making the original material "user-friendly," as well as Barbara Watkins, Senior Editor, and Anna Brackett, Senior Production Editor, at The Guilford Press. I wish to extend my appreciation to Victoria Russell, Eileen Stuart-Shor, the late Richard Friedman, Ann Webster, and Jay Galipeault for their support and words of encouragement over the years. Finally, a special thanks is owed to the peer advisors who have shared their experiences and support with the hundreds of patients who followed in their footsteps.

Preface
to the Revised Edition

To heal does not necessarily imply to cure. It can simply mean helping people to achieve a way of life compatible with their individual aspirations—to restore their freedom to make choices—even in the presence of continuing disease.
—*René Dubos,* Human Nature *(1978)*

Chronic pain is an incurable problem for millions of people around the world, and yet there is reason for hope: The health sciences continue their important work to understand, treat, and eventually prevent chronic pain, and the map of the human genome promises dramatic future insights into chronic pain syndromes. What is available for you who are suffering with chronic pain right now is to treat your symptoms and learn to live as best you can with the pain. You still wish to be cured, of course, but until there is a cure, you can learn how to help yourself feel better in spite of the pain. Recent research led by my colleague Dr. Paul Arnstein shows the importance of self-efficacy—of feeling empowered. Having the skills to manage, function, and cope with pain—the skills taught in this book—is proven to reduce disability and depression. As one of my patients once said, "I know I'm going to have a good day because I know how to make it a good day." When you have a chronic problem, be it diabetes, heart disease, or chronic pain, the benefits of knowing what can and can't be done cannot be underestimated. If you suffer from chronic pain, I urge you to become a full partner with your health professional in managing your symptoms.

This revised edition of *Managing Pain Before It Manages You* is updated to include current ideas about chronic pain and treatment. Recommendations for using drugs for chronic pain have changed since the first edition, and I have updated those in Chapter 2, "Understanding Pain." In Chapter 4, "The Body–Mind Connection," I emphasize the importance of maintaining activities inside and outside the home. In Chapter 5, "The Power of the Mind," I have included practical suggestions on anger management, journaling, and how to change negative self-talk. I have extensively updated Chapter 7, "Nutrition and Pain," to include information on the American Heart Association's dietary recommendations released in October 2000. Information is also included on the newest research on omega-3 fatty acids to decrease inflammation. In Chapter 9, "Effective Problem Solving," I offer more on how to accomplish your personal goals. In Chapter 10, "The End of the Beginning," I've added guidance on how best to manage a future pain flare-up. I have also added a new appendix, "Complementary Alternative Medicine." It provides a description of common alternative therapies used for pain treatment. Finally, I have greatly expanded the information in the "Letter to Health Care Professionals" to encourage and support the dialogue between the client/patient in pain and the health care professional as well as the adaptation of material in this book to clients/patients at various stages of willingness to change.

My colleagues and I have almost 20 years of experience using the techniques described in this book; tens of thousands of patients have used the program. The book has been translated into Spanish, Portuguese, Polish, and Chinese, and an audiotape has been made. In my travels nationally and internationally, I have been struck by the usefulness of this treatment across many different cultures and pain problems. The skills in this book are helpful whether the pain comes from work injuries or from disease. The skills can be learned in groups or individually, in pain clinics, independent psychotherapy, primary care, and physical therapy. Transcending these differences, the challenges in living, working, and loving in spite of the pain are similar. This program can assist people in meeting those common challenges. This book may not be for everyone in chronic pain, but if you or someone you love is in chronic pain and needs assistance, I encourage you to read on.

Before You Begin
How This Book Can Help You

Thank God, I finally realized that pain may be mandatory, but suffering is optional . . .

—*Craig T. Nelson, actor*

This book has been carefully developed from years of work with brave people experiencing pain. If you have begun reading this book, you have probably been living with pain for some time. You may have a painful disease for which there is no cure, or you may be among those who have experienced the tremendous frustration of trying to explain to doctors that your pain is real and it is persisting, even though they can identify no cause for it. In spite of your protests, they may tell you that all your tests have come back negative, that there is no medical explanation for your continued suffering, that surgery should have worked, or something similar. They may also suggest, directly or indirectly, that your condition is the result of emotional stress—or perhaps even that "it's all in your head"—and that you should consider seeing a psychologist.

As if this weren't bad enough, you must return home and face your anxious loved ones, who have been hoping against hope for a "miracle cure" so that you and they can resume something like normal family life. You must now tell them that your condition is unchanged and that you have exhausted all medical help. If you have not returned to work but run into colleagues, you must explain to them that you have not been on vacation and politely tolerate their unsupportive comments ("Aren't you better *yet*?") or their suggestions for home remedies (snake livers, copper bracelets, etc.). In short, you may feel abandoned, panicky, and utterly alone.

This book is for you if you can say, "I have chronic pain, it's real, and I need help." But you don't have to be at the end of your rope to use this book. The skills it describes can also help you get more out of your ongoing medical treatment. For you at this time, pain may be mandatory, but suffering is optional. And you are definitely not alone.

This book is also for you if you are the relative or friend of a person in chronic pain. It may increase your own understanding of the pain experience, or it could be an important gift to that special person. Finally, this book is for you if you are a health care professional; it can be a valuable resource for you and your patients who must live in pain.

Is the following story familiar to you?

A Common Story

Pat entered the new specialist's office, tired and apprehensive at the prospect of describing her pain once again to a stranger. No one ever seemed to listen when she tried to explain what it was like to wake up and go to bed day after day in pain. Every day it became more of an effort to take care of herself and her family. Her children wondered, "Gee, Mom, what's wrong with you? Why won't they fix it?" Two nights ago her husband—frustrated, she knew, at his own sense of powerlessness—had snapped, "Why can't you just ignore it?" She remembered her family physician's words at her last visit: "There is nothing else I can do. You have chronic pain and must learn to live with it." She had cried all the way home. Her doctor, however, had also given her the name of a pain specialist who worked with people in chronic pain and had been successful in helping them. She didn't like this alternative at all. But after spending thousands of dollars, experiencing medication side effects, undergoing unsuccessful surgery, and seeing six consultants, she was no closer to getting rid of the pain.

So now here she was waiting for someone else to give her bad news. The pain management doctor, however, asked types of questions she had not heard before—questions about her experience of pain: Had she ever noticed that her pain increased with certain activities, particularly when she ignored the early spasms warning her to stop? Did she find that if she was anxious or upset about family or financial matters, her pain flared up as well? Was she more short-tempered than she used to be? Did she cry more easily? Was she experiencing non-pain symptoms—like shortness of breath, palpitations, fatigue, or sleep problems? Pat answered yes to all of these questions.

The pain specialist told Pat that her pain was real—it was absolutely not "all in her head"—but that medical science did not yet know how to take it away. She was one of millions of people caught in a tangled web of chronic pain. However, many of Pat's symptoms were manageable, because they were the results of ignoring the limits placed on her by the pain. By identifying new ways of working with and relating to her pain, she could feel less helpless, less hopeless, and more in control. She could even feel more productive and better about herself just by practicing certain techniques and modifying her daily routine in a way that allowed her to take her discomfort into consideration. The threads of Pat's pain web could in fact be untangled and rewoven into a safety net if she followed this program.

Pat was still a little skeptical, but she decided to give it a try. She felt that at this point she had nothing to lose and everything to gain.

This book describes the program that helped Pat. It can help you too.

How Effective Is the Program?

Like Pat, are you still a little skeptical?

The program presented in this book has been proven effective in helping people in chronic pain improve their quality of life. My colleagues and I first reported this in a paper published in the scientific journal *The Clinical Journal of Pain* (7: 305–310, 1991).

We found that before participating in a pain management program identical to the one presented here, our patients averaged 12 doctor visits a year. After participating, the patients did not need to see their doctors as frequently (down to seven visits per year), and doctor visits remained decreased for up to two years following the termination of the program. Furthermore, the patients reported decreases in their depression, their anxiety, their pain's severity, and their pain's interference in their activities. They also noted increases in their feelings of being in control and in their general activity levels.

My colleagues and I believe that the program works as the direct result of helping people with chronic pain increase their ability to manage, function, and cope with pain. This belief in the ability to manage, function, and cope with challenges is called "self-efficacy." Our more recent research published in the journal *Pain* (81: 483–491, 1999) has shown that whether or not you believe you can do these things influences how much you are depressed or disabled by your pain. Developing this ability to manage, function, and cope with your pain will help you gain control over the pain, and practicing the skills in this book will help you develop that ability.

What Can You Expect?

The program described here does not offer any "miracle cures." It also does not promise to make your life exactly the way it was before you had the pain. However, no one is suggesting that you should just passively endure your pain. If you learn the skills and apply the techniques presented in this book, you can expect to become active and involved in your life again, in a way that will minimize pain increases and reduce the distress of having a pain problem. By becoming involved in your pain treatment, you become part of the solution to the problem.

What's Involved?

This pain management program will help you understand what chronic pain is and why certain treatments may have been prescribed for you in the past. You will be asked to explore your pain experience by tracking it on a daily basis, using a diary to record and compare the effects on your pain of doing things differently. This is a way of beginning to untangle the pain web you have been caught in. You will be given many opportunities to reflect on how you wish to live each day. You will be encouraged to consider that many old habits that served you well in the past may not work now that you are challenged by pain.

Many ways to reduce stress will be presented. These will include breath exercises, techniques that bring about a particular physical reaction called the "relaxation response," stretching techniques, and body awareness exercises. In addition, you will be shown how to become more active with less pain by learning how to pace and plan your daily activities. Methods of moving when you are in pain and using breathing to reduce the tension of pain during movement will be explored. Ways of using nutrition to your advantage will also be discussed.

Moreover, skills for coping with the sadness, anxiety, or anger you may be experiencing will be taught. In many instances, these emotions are the results of the expectations and beliefs you held before the pain came into your life. Methods for communicating your needs clearly and expressing yourself effectively to those around you, including your health care provider, will also be described. Finally, problem-solving techniques and ways to begin planning a new life in spite of the pain will be shared. You will then be ready to reweave the untangled threads of your old pain web into a safety net.

This program is meant to empower you to act in your own best interests. In fact, by deciding to read this far, you have been learning to exercise choice. You may at any time put down this book and stop the process, but choosing to go on can open many doors for you. Will you stay where you are, feeling trapped and misunderstood, or will you begin to evaluate and understand how your pain can be modified? Will you continue to feel that you are at the mercy of your pain, or will you begin to live with hope? You do have choices.

How to Use This Book

This program has been used by many people who feel just like you do. They have, like you, bravely made the first step toward managing their pain by picking up this book. Whether you are reading it by yourself or with a group of other people in pain, you can be assured that your struggles are universal ones. Reading the patients' stories presented throughout the book may also help you to feel less lonely in your work.

Most people find that they make the best use of the book by reading about a chapter a week, but everyone should set his or her own pace. Allow enough time to answer all the questions in each chapter and complete all the exploration tasks (see the next section). More skills and techniques will be added as you read through the book. Many of the tasks do not require you to make extra time in your schedule for them; they simply require you to pay attention to how you do the things you already do. Some of the skills and techniques, such as the ones in the chapters on attitudes and communication, may take a little more time.

Keep in mind that there is no need for you to finish all 10 chapters in 10 weeks. Research studies with self-changers and smokers suggest that it takes at least 10 weeks to begin to change behavior and that six months of sustained action are required to progress to maintenance of these changes. Research has also shown that real change and therefore real benefits take place only when people act upon the written word. If you are really in doubt about the benefits of working with this book, just reading it may be what you need to do at this time. If you are ready to change the way you are feeling and to improve on your life in pain, however, then actually carrying out the exercises in this book is essential.

Special Features of the Book

A number of special features have been provided in this book to help you. These include chapter summaries, exploration tasks, supplementary reading lists, appendices, and end-of-book worksheets and other materials.

A summary of each chapter is given at the chapter's end. Reading the summary first may be helpful in grasping the highlights of each chapter—a preview of coming attractions, so to speak. Reviewing the summary after reading the chapter is useful for picking up certain points or aspects that you may have forgotten.

Exploration tasks are included in most chapters, and each set of tasks should be completed before you move on to the next chapter. These tasks are designed to reinforce what you've learned in the chapter by having you apply the skills and techniques to your particular situation and put them into practice. They will take you from the level of theory to the level of action, where the real learning is done. If you are working on a chapter a week, the exploration tasks will clarify what skills you should be practicing at any particular time.

There are supplementary reading lists at the end of most chapters. The contents of these lists (and a few additional resources) are presented in bibliography form in Appendix D. You can use this reading material to help you develop your coping skills further.

Appendix A, "Common Chronic Pain Conditions," is a review of observations I have made on various chronic pain syndromes. It can serve as a resource for support groups or for further treatment recommendations in some instances. Appendix B, "Complementary Alternative Medicine," discusses other therapies used for pain treatment. Appendix C, "Working Comfortably," was written by a former patient to help those who must work at a computer terminal. It has important recommendations to prevent injuries or relapses.

At the end of the book, following the index, are worksheets and other materials that can be photocopied by purchasers of this book for personal use only (see copyright page for details). To faciliate photocopying, one set has been perforated and can be easily removed. The worksheets include a pain diary sheet (see Chapter 1 for an explanation of its use); a relaxation response diary sheet (see Chapter 3); an increasing activities worksheet (see Chapter 4); a food diary sheet (see Chapter 7); a worksheet for monitoring your self-talk, emotions, and other responses to stressful events (see Chapter 5); and a feedback sheet for giving your health care professional information about your pain experience (see Chapter 8).

Additional materials include (1) a "Do Not Disturb" sign that can be copied and hung on your door to prevent interruptions during your practice of relaxation response techniques; and (2) a letter to your health care professional, which I encourage you to copy and share with him or her on your next visit. It explains how he or she can help you use the information in this book and helps enlist him or her if you have picked up the book on your own.

A Final Note

The solutions offered in this book are for real people living in the real world. The skills and techniques are practical, and the recommendations are based on years of working with people in pain just like you. You are encouraged to read and reread carefully even statements that you may find disagreeable or distressful. The assertion that it is possible to live in pain or that after reading this book you will not necessarily be pain-free may be the last thing you want to hear. I do understand that it is not your choice to be in pain and that your life has been changed by your pain. These recommendations for working with your pain and rebuilding your life are not made lightly. They are made because I have seen that, with help, people are able to live with and even rise above their pain in remarkable ways. You can be productive, can enjoy life's pleasures, and can even fulfill some dreams if you apply what you read in this book to your pain problem. I hope that this will be a positive new beginning for you. Welcome to the program!

Chapter 1

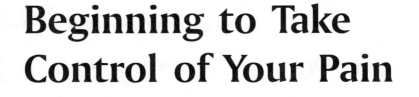

Beginning to Take Control of Your Pain

You may still have doubts about whether you can ever enjoy life again while you are in chronic pain or whether life will ever be worth living with chronic pain. Nevertheless, let's at least explore how living a life of quality with chronic pain is possible. The keys are to take responsibility for your pain (not in the sense of accepting blame for it yourself or assigning blame to others, but in the sense of accepting "ownership" of it); to determine exactly what your problems are as a result of the pain; and to reassess your goals in the light of this information. This chapter gives you your first set of tools for beginning to take control of your pain: diary keeping and goal setting. To begin, look at the first of the three keys: accepting ownership of your pain.

Accepting Ownership of Your Pain

As you define it at this moment, your problem is that you are in pain and the pain won't go away. This is an important first step; before you can do anything about your pain, you need to acknowledge that it exists. However, you may also feel inclined at this point to blame others for your pain. You may feel that your doctors have failed you by not finding and curing the source of the pain or at least for not making you feel better. You may believe that your loved ones are not doing anything to help you or are showing a lack of understanding or empathy about your problem. You may even feel that society is to blame for causing the situation that put you in pain in the first place or for not making it easier for you to seek help.

The fact that you may be sad, angry, or anxious about the disruption of your whole life as a result of the pain experience is both understandable and normal. Under these circumstances, it may be very tempting to feel that others are to blame for the pain and ought to be responsible for taking it away. Indeed, many people in pain put their whole lives on hold waiting for others—their physicians, their families, or society—to do just this. The difficulty with this, however, is that wanting to give away both the pain and the responsibility for it will only prolong and contribute to your feelings of powerlessness. If your pain is not going away any time soon—and this is the very nature of chronic pain— then taking upon yourself the responsibility for living with it may begin to return control of your life to you. If you can adopt an attitude of "ownership" of the pain problem, you have the potential for gaining the upper hand over it. Although you may need assistance from your health care professional, your family, and society in untangling yourself from your pain web, gathering the threads together and reweaving them into a safety net for yourself is ultimately your task and yours alone.

What you may now be thinking is something like this: "Oh, great. So I'm responsible for my pain, huh? I'm to blame? That's what everybody's been saying—or at least hinting—all along. I feel bad and guilty enough as it is." That is not what is meant here at all. As you probably already know, self-blame and guilt can be paralyzing emotions. They can make you feel that because you are such a bad and worthless person, there's no point in doing anything at all. Accepting ownership of your pain, on the other hand, means acknowledging that you *are* a worthwhile person, that there *is* a point in doing something, and that you *do* have choices. It is very different from blaming yourself.

Chronic pain is complex, with numerous origins and treatments, and is grossly misunderstood. This book will provide you with the information you need to move forward. Even though your life will be different from the way it was before you developed the pain, you can change some aspects of the pain, and can learn to accept or work with other aspects so that they cause you less distress. Your task will be difficult—but not impossible.

Determining Exactly What Your Problems Are

> Order and simplification are the first steps toward mastery of a subject— the actual enemy is the unknown.
> —*Thomas Mann,* The Magic Mountain *(1924)*

The Importance of Tracking Your Pain Levels

One important way to gain control over your pain is to record it so that you can see how certain factors—for instance, activities, the weather, tension, and sleeplessness—

increase or decrease your pain levels. This should be done three times a day, at regular times that are convenient for you. For example, you might record your pain level when you awaken, after lunch, and then again at bedtime. Such consistency is important, because if you record your pain only when you are aware of it, you won't necessarily feel it at the times when your pain is altered. Recording the pain at regular intervals will allow you to detect over time whether there are any patterns to your pain experience. These patterns should permit you to determine the exact nature of your problems more easily.

Many people are resistant to the idea of recording their pain, and you may be one of them. Not only are you in pain to begin with, but it's an additional hassle to have to record all this stuff—and three times a day! "Why do I have to do this? It's not fair!" you may say. Perhaps the following story will help.

Paula was very angry at the thought of recording her pain levels. Her back hurt and she already knew she was in pain. Why did she have to write it down three times every day? She didn't have time for such a ridiculous activity.

At first, Paula was so miserable that recording the pain just made her realize how bad she felt. Gradually, she realized how much she had denied the pain in her back and how it prevented her from doing anything productive or pleasurable. Not only had she had to give up working outside the home, but also she barely kept up with the household chores. Her house certainly wasn't as clean as it used to be. Even worse, she was irritable toward her husband and yelled at her children. She rarely saw her friends and really didn't care any more about going out. Somehow this just wasn't the way Paula wanted to live.

Paula also began to see how she pushed herself throughout the day and then collapsed at night. Her back was stiff when she awoke, and the pain gradually increased during the day. What was causing it? Was she not pacing herself? Was she stressed by her routine? Slowly, the answers became clear.

Over time, Paula saw that recording her pain helped her learn more about the relationship her pain had with what she did and how she did it. She was able to incorporate the skills she learned in the pain management program into her daily routine and was eventually able to bring the pain much more under her control.

If you don't think that recording your pain will be a chore, that's great. If you do, consider this: You have done your best in your current situation, and it still hasn't been effective in controlling your pain. Recording your pain levels can help you determine where you might be stuck and point you in the right direction. You can't count on remembering exactly what your pain feels like under all conditions over a long period of time. So give the recording method a shot—it just might work for you. Remember: *What you know, you can master.*

Keeping a Pain Diary

An effective way of recording your pain is to use the pain diary worksheet that is provided at the end of this book. There is a sample of a completed pain diary form, along with a blank pain diary form that can be copied.

Instructions

In the pain diary, it is important that you differentiate between the physical sensation of the pain and any negative emotional response to the pain. "Physical sensation" refers, for example, to the achiness, stabbing, burning, pounding, tightness, and other physical sensations you may feel. "Emotional response" refers to the negative experience of pain and is a measure of the suffering—for example, the frustration, anxiety, anger, or sadness— you may feel.

Note that the word "feel" can be used to describe both physical/body sensations and emotional/mind reactions. This dual meaning can give rise to confusion when you try to describe the pain experience to yourself and to the outside world. I began asking patients to make the physical sensation/emotional response distinction years ago when I noticed that at the last session of the pain group they were talking about how great they felt, and yet their pain recordings were only decreased a little from the beginning of the program. I was puzzled by this, so I asked them to explain it. They responded without hesitation: "We still have the pain [the physical sensation], but we *feel* so much better about it [the emotional response]. We aren't so helpless. We know what to do about our pain, and we feel in control again."

Much can be done about your level of emotional response to the pain. You can begin by getting in touch with how you experience your pain, both physically and emotionally. You may find that either the physical *or* the emotional feelings predominate; it will take some time for you to make the distinction. Some of the exercises in the next few chapters will help you to separate these feelings.

1. Record your pain level on the pain diary form three times a day at regular intervals, as described previously—for example, morning, noon, and bedtime.
2. On the diary sheet there is a space to describe the situation for each physical sensation/emotional response rating. For example, were you watching TV, eating lunch, sitting at a computer, or fixing dinner? Note what activity you were engaged in at the time.
3. Rate your physical sensation and your emotional response separately by using numbers to represent physical intensity and decreased activities and emotional intensity. The numbers you give to your physical sensation and emotional response do not necessarily have to increase or decrease together. For example, you can have a high level of pain sensation and yet not necessarily suffer emotionally because of it. This will become more apparent as you proceed through the book and learn new pain management skills. Give ratings on a scale from 0 to 10 as follows:

Ratings	Physical sensation/activities	Emotional response
0	No painful physical sensation No alteration in activities	No negative emotional response
1–4	Low intensity of physical sensation, minimal effect on activities	Minimal/low level of negative emotions
5–6	Moderate intensity of physical sensation associated with increased body tension; moderate restriction of activities	Moderate intensity of negative emotions
7–8	Significant pain sensation associated with difficulty moving; decreased activities	Significant negative emotions, making it hard to engage in activities
9–10	Severe pain sensation associated with inability to move; able to participate in only minimal activities; bedridden	Severe depression, anxiety, or despair associated with significant impairment of thinking

It may take several weeks to establish what the numbers mean for you. This is quite normal. Pain is a personal experience, and you'll only be rating your own experience. (If you have particular or continuing difficulty, however, see the "Rating Your Pain" exercise under "Listening to Your Body" in Chapter 4.)

4. At the end of each day, add the numbers from the three ratings for physical sensation together and average them by dividing the total by three so that you have one daily physical sensation rating. Do the same for your ratings of emotional response. Making a graph of the numbers for different times of day and for the daily averages can help you see the pain patterns more clearly over the weeks and months during which you develop your program of self-management. I recommend that you continue to fill out the pain diary form for at least three months. You can stop once your pain levels appear stable and you are feeling better and in more control of your response to the pain. You can always start again should your pain worsen or a new symptom occur.

5. There is also a place to record any medication or action you took to help alleviate the pain. For example, if you soaked in a hot tub, went for a walk, stretched, or took two aspirins, record the fact.

The pain diary is intended for your benefit and self-exploration. Therefore, if you find it more helpful to record pain in two separate areas of the body or would like to differentiate emotional responses to pain from emotional responses to life, you are encouraged to do so. The pain diary can also be an important source of information when you see your health care professional, particularly when the two of you are tracking your treatment responses or symptom flare-ups.

Noting Variations in Your Pain

If you find yourself rating your physical sensation with the same number three times a day, seven days a week, examine your pain more closely. Physical sensation and emotional responses vary; they rarely remain constant for days and weeks at a time. It is common, however, for people in pain to think of their pain as overwhelming and self-absorbing, unvarying and unremitting.

The natural variation in physical sensation and emotional response is the result of attention shifting from one thing to another, compounded by additional factors such as mood, fatigue, or muscle tension, which influence the pain experience from moment to moment. The brain, the final judge of sensory and emotional input, tends to pay the most attention to changing levels of sensation or events. It quickly becomes bored with constant stimulation, sounds, pain, and so forth, whether from outside or inside the body. Therefore, pain and the awareness of pain vary as well.

For example, if you are in a room with a fan, you may be aware of the sound when you first enter the room; after a short period of time, however, you will "forget" its presence. If it shuts off, you may pay attention again to the absence of the sound for a few seconds. Likewise, you may not be aware of the pressure of your back against a chair as you sit reading this, but now that I've pointed it out, you are suddenly aware of it. This awareness, too, will suddenly disappear after a few seconds as you read on.

You can make use of the brain's short span of attention to constant stimulation as a means of altering the pain experience. Such techniques will be discussed in later chapters.

What's Next?

You are most likely going to feel worse for the next few weeks. You may say, "Oh, no! I thought this program was supposed to make me feel better, not worse." Well, don't panic just yet. This program begins by helping you identify what you have been experiencing, both physically and emotionally. If you begin to feel worse, it is not because the pain itself is getting worse, but because you are bringing it into consciousness, and this alters your perception. Remember this for future reference: Changing your awareness changes the pain experience.

Most people use denial to cope with their pain. This may work for short-term problems. Long-term problems usually require conscious action. Conscious action allows you to engage in activities in a way that will not make your pain worse. You will be asked to increase your consciousness or awareness of your daily thoughts, experiences, and interactions throughout this program. You will learn how to distract yourself from the pain; however, this will be a conscious action on your part, completely under your control, and free from any harmful side effects. It is a process, which means that it takes time, and you are now just beginning it.

Setting Goals

Many times people in pain report feeling scattered, adrift, unfocused, and unsuccessful. These symptoms are in part a result of unfulfilled expectations, because pain restricts activities and function. At present, no doubt, you find yourself unable to accomplish and do all that you had hoped. The ability to function and engage in meaningful activity gives meaning to life. When meaningful activity is apparently taken away because of chronic pain, you suffer even more. Diary keeping is one way of bringing focus to your life by bringing order and simplification to this "big unknown," the pain), and determining what can be done to minimize or cope with it.

Another way to gain some control over your pain is by setting goals through which you can slowly bring order, success, and accomplishment back to your life. In this particular instance, setting goals will serve you by helping you commit yourself to this program. But if you are not used to setting goals, it can be tricky. The key is to set *achievable* goals—that is, ones that can be accomplished. This is particularly important when you are learning how to live with your pain, because you don't need to feel like a failure any more than you perhaps already do. There are ways to set goals so that you cannot fail. When you take the goal-setting process slowly and easily, with each small success you can reach to higher challenges.

Let's start by considering three goals that you would like to achieve through working with the material in this book. The goals should be short-term ones that can be accomplished in two to three months.

Goal-Setting Criteria

Use the following criteria to develop your goals:

1. *A goal should be measurable.* Can you evaluate when the goal has been reached?
2. *A goal should be realistic.* Is it possible to achieve, even in pain?
3. *A goal should be behavioral.* Does it involve specific actions or steps to take?
4. *A goal should be "I"-centered.* Are *you* the one engaging in the actions or behaviors to be measured?
5. *A goal should be desirable.* Do you want the outcome enough to put forth the effort?

> Cindy's goal was to feel less stressed in four weeks. It sounded reasonable, but what exactly did it mean? Was the goal "feeling less stressed" measurable? What was "feeling stressed"? What did she mean by "less stressed"? What behavior change in the form of specific actions or steps would Cindy need to engage in to accomplish this goal? Her success would be left to chance if she didn't answer
>
> *(cont.)*

these questions. And leaving it to chance would not guarantee her success; it might even make it unlikely.

Cindy reworked her goal and decided that to her, "feeling stressed" meant feeling tense in the back of her neck. She wanted to be able to control the tension in her neck. If she could do that, maybe her headaches would be helped too. Now she could make a list of behaviors through which she could accomplish her *measurable* and *desirable* goal—decreased tension in the neck and a decrease in the number of headaches.

Cindy decided that she would swim three times a week, take a stretch break from her work at the computer every hour for 60 seconds (see Chapter 4), and practice a relaxation response technique (see Chapter 3) once a day. She thus made her goal *behavioral* (these were specific, clear steps to take), *realistic* (these steps would be relatively easy to take), and *"I"-centered* (she, not someone else, would be engaging in these activities).

After Cindy had worked toward her goal for a while, she could see for herself whether the tension was decreased in her neck and whether this was influencing her headaches. Her success was not left to chance but was the result of a conscious effort on her part.

Goal-Setting Exercise

Now list three goals related to working with this pain management program that you would like to accomplish in the next two to three months. Make them achievable in each of the five ways previously described.

Let's use Cindy's goal as an example:

1. **Goal:** *Decrease tension in the back of the neck and decrease headaches.*

   Steps to take to reach that goal:

   A. *Swim three times a week.*

   B. *Take frequent stretch breaks at the computer.*

   C. *Practice a relaxation response technique once a day.*

Now it's your turn.

1. **Goal:** _____

   Steps to take to reach that goal:

   A. _____

   B. _____

   C. _____

2. Goal: _____

Steps to take to reach that goal:

A. _____

B. _____

C. _____

3. Goal: _____

Steps to take to reach that goal:

A. _____

B. _____

C. _____

Setting goals at this time is a way of making a commitment to this self-management program. If you find yourself confused or resistant, ask yourself why. Have you been clear enough in defining what you want? Do you want something that you can't achieve at this time? Is there a way you can modify the desire and make it achievable? Don't be surprised if you find yourself feeling sad, angry, or frustrated with this exercise, particularly if there are things you wish to do but can't. The ability to be flexible and identify other goals that are available to you, in spite of the pain, can be very rewarding. Once again, you do have choices. Setting goals is a step toward identifying those options.

Congratulate yourself for having the courage and determination to begin this process and to gain new understanding of and control over your life!

Summary

- Taking ownership of your pain is the first step toward gaining control over it.
- Recording your pain helps you see what factors increase or decrease it and thus exactly what your problems are.
- The pain diary helps you track your pain sensation and emotional response.
- Acknowledging your pain may make you feel worse . . . temporarily. However, you can learn to distract yourself consciously from pain.
- Setting achievable goals—that is, ones that are measurable, realistic, behavioral, "I"-centered, and desirable—is important to success.

Exploration Tasks

1. When your pain gets worse, list the things that you do now to make it better:

_____

_____

_____

_____

2. Draw a picture of you and your pain here. Use crayons or colored pencils. No black-and-white pictures, please! This artwork will not be displayed, but it can be an important exercise to look at pain in a nonverbal way.

Use this space to draw yourself and your pain:

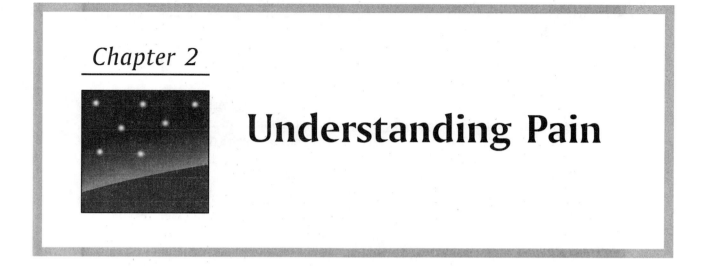

Chapter 2

Understanding Pain

Pain, like fever, is a symptom. It is also a vital component of the human experience. Let's take a look at the various meanings of pain:

- *Biologically,* pain is a signal that the body has been harmed.
- *Psychologically,* pain is experienced as emotional suffering.
- *Behaviorally,* pain alters the way a person moves and acts.
- *Cognitively,* pain calls for thinking about its meaning, its cause, and possible remedies.
- *Spiritually,* pain has been a reminder of mortality.
- *Culturally,* pain has been used to test people's fortitude or to force their submission.

Pain is a complex process, and the pain signal can be magnified, minimized, and reinterpreted by a person's experiences.

Categories of Pain

The body experiences two categories of pain: "acute pain" and "chronic pain."

Acute Pain

Acute pain warns us of tissue injury or harm. It can be associated with trauma (abnormal crush, stretch, or tear of tissue) or inflammation (in response to infection, injury, or disease). Acute pain is time limited and lasts long enough for healing to begin, generally from 24 hours to 10 days. Here are some of the circumstances associated with acute pain:

- *A burn.* We touch the hot iron, and instantly the hand is withdrawn. The hot iron has stimulated pain receptors in the hand. It is too much heat for the tissue to be exposed to safely. A reflex to move the hand out of harm's way occurs automatically, and then we rush to the sink to run cool water over the burned area.
- *Appendicitis.* The pain from an infected appendix is a more complicated process because it involves inflammation in an internal organ, the appendix. At first the person with appendicitis may be aware only of a vague stomachache in the area around the belly button. Appetite may decrease or fever may be present. As the appendix becomes more inflamed, the pain is localized to the right lower quadrant of the abdomen, and the muscles above the appendix spasm. The pain serves as a warning that something is wrong and drives a person to search for relief, usually through surgical removal of the appendix.
- *Labor pains.* The pain during childbirth is caused by stretching of the cervix around the baby's head and contractions of the uterine muscle. Although the pain receptors in the cervix respond to the abnormal stretching, the woman's experience of labor pain can be modified by distraction, massage, and supportive coaching and by blocking the pain pathways with anesthetics.

In all of these examples, pain is a warning symptom that triggers a person to act. These behaviors can be automatic, such as pulling the hand away from the hot iron, or purposeful, such as seeking help. Anxiety and fear are normal emotional responses to pain that further motivate a person to seek relief. But the situation may modify these emotional responses. Modified emotions, in turn, can modify the experience of the pain, as seen in the labor pain of childbirth. Acute pain is an important symptom to heed. But once treatment begins there is no advantage to withholding pain relief. Unrelieved pain after surgery can cause complications (pneumonia and immobility), and in patients with cancer it can cause unnecessary suffering. Supporting these observations is a major education initiative in the United States to advocate for timely and adequate treatment of acute and cancer pain.

Chronic Pain

Chronic pain is different. Like a broken fire alarm clanging when there is no fire, chronic pain may persist without a good reason. The symptom of pain, originally a warning, now becomes the problem. It doesn't go away.

Some chronic pain problems may be the result of ongoing (chronic) inflammation (rheumatoid arthritis) or nerve damage (diabetic neuropathy, radiation neuritis). Chronic pain often has an ill-defined source or cause, lasts longer than three months, and is commonly associated with multiple biological, psychological, and sociological consequences.

Here are some problems associated with chronic pain:

- Back or neck pain
- Interstitial cystitis
- Diabetic neuropathy
- Osteoarthritis
- Fibromyalgia
- Pelvic pain
- Post-shingles pain

A variation of chronic pain is chronic intermittent pain. That is, pain-free times alternate with weeks or even months of daily pain. Examples of chronic intermittent pain include migraine headaches, cluster headaches, and irritable bowel syndrome.

The Experience of Chronic Pain

With chronic pain, the pain experience may be magnified because of the long duration of the symptoms with no relief. This experience may be modified by the environment (changes in weather), expectations ("If I have pain, I must be doing something wrong"), a search for meaning ("Why me?"), and/or cultural beliefs ("No pain, no gain"). Your perceptions (beliefs, attitudes, moods) greatly affect your experience of chronic pain.

Although there may be no clear explanation for your chronic pain, you are understandably driven biologically and psychologically to resolve the problem. Remember that the presence of pain and the pressure to act on its presence are established in a very old and primitive part of the brain. When the pain system is doing its job, it is a warning of danger and harm. When the system is overloaded or has begun reacting indiscriminately, it can be a source of physical and emotional stress. As a result, you may suffer even more symptoms (such as fatigue, muscle tension, and insomnia). These additional symptoms are the result of the stress you suffer from chronic pain.

For months or years, you have been experiencing the constant stimulus of pain. Biologically, you have had to live with a signal that usually requires the utmost urgency and attention. Psychologically, you may feel anxious, depressed, and abandoned. Behaviorally, you may have become less sociable; you may have withdrawn from activities or the company of others. Cognitively, you may think yourself inadequate to meet this challenge, or you may be at your wits' end not knowing what to do. Spiritually, you may feel beaten down and abandoned. And culturally, you may be fighting beliefs or expectations of how you should suffer.

It's important for you to understand what chronic pain is and isn't and what the mechanisms for keeping it going are thought to be. Your enemy is the unknown. Understanding the pain process can bring you closer to its mastery. You can begin to do that by keeping a pain diary, which helps you establish what the pain experience is like for you.

Now that you've had a chance to learn a little about acute and chronic pain, take a minute to read the following. This is a story common to many who end up with chronic pain. See whether you can identify both the acute and chronic phases of the process.

Sarah was a very active 31-year-old English professor who liked to garden, dance, and ride horses in her spare time. One day as she bent to turn her compost pile, she experienced searing pain down her right leg, causing her to limp as she walked away. She took it easy for a week, stopped exercising, and didn't ride her horses to see whether the pain would get better. It didn't. She then went to her doctor. An examination showed that Sarah had lost the reflexes in her right leg. A computerized axial tomography (CAT) scan revealed a herniated disc in her lower back. She was referred to a neurosurgeon, who recommended surgery.

By now Sarah's pain was constantly sending knife-like sensations into her leg and down the calf to her foot. It was impossible for her to find a comfortable position in which to sleep, and the constant pain was always on her mind. She had nightmares of having surgery and being confined to a wheelchair for the rest of her life. She was anxious and frightened. She took a medical leave of absence from her job because the pain would not allow her to carry out her teaching responsibilities.

Sarah spent three anxious and painful weeks hoping that the pain would subside; when it didn't, she made the decision to have the surgery. It went well, and even though Sarah was sore and tight from the incision, her leg was already feeling better than it had in weeks. The pain from her incision was made tolerable by pain medication. She was able to walk out of the hospital in three days, and within eight weeks she was back at work. In addition, she was able to garden, ride her horse, and even dance without experiencing pain.

Two months later Sarah began experiencing pain in her right knee; she attributed this to a recent hiking trip. Again, she waited for the pain to go away on its own. After two weeks, she started noticing that she was constantly rubbing her back, particularly at the end of the day. Also, she was waking up in the middle of the night with painful back spasms. Her anxiety about having another herniated disc created more sleep disturbance. She went back to the neurosurgeon, who found nothing abnormal upon examination and recommended waiting a few more weeks to see whether the pain would improve. But it increased, and Sarah stopped doing anything requiring physical effort.

Once again she returned to the neurosurgeon, who performed magnetic resonance imagery (MRI) with gadolinium; this revealed nothing abnormal, except for some increased scar tissue around the previous laminectomy site. Because it did not appear to press on the nerve roots and wasn't operable, the surgeon wondered whether Sarah had been under any stress lately. He recommended that she keep busy with her life and suggested that the problem would resolve itself in time. Sarah left his office in a daze. By the time she got home, her imagination was running wild. "I'm in pain. Why can't they find something? What if they missed something important?" Sarah thought about her aunt, who had had back pain and was told nothing was wrong; the aunt eventually died of cancer.

Sarah felt terrified and desperate. She could no longer do normal things around the house. Vacuuming was agonizing. Standing or sitting for any extended time was painful. Her patience with her students was becoming short, and she began to miss days at work. She was generally too tired to socialize; even when she did, she felt as though she was always complaining. After a period of time, her friends stopped calling. She felt exhausted, alone, defective, miserable, and unlovable. She no longer had control over her body. The pain was in control now.

One day Sarah decided she should be able to do what she needed to do in spite of the pain. She was tough; all she needed to do was push through her daily activities. She cleaned the house, taught her classes, and took a dozen aspirin that day to help keep the pain down. The next morning, she couldn't get out of bed.

Sarah then went to another surgeon, who ordered a myelogram. The test revealed no herniated disc, but the surgeon suggested that stabilizing the spine by a fusion would give her relief. Sarah was so desperate that she had the operation. But it didn't work, and the pain just continued. She became even more depressed. By now she was unable to work. Her disability insurance supplied some sustenance, but her income certainly was not the same as when she was working. Furthermore, the disability insurance representatives were harassing her with paperwork, which necessitated more trips to the various doctors to fill out the forms. The office staff members made her feel like a pest. The doctors never filled out the paperwork on time, and she always panicked at the end of the month if the check was late.

Sarah's family doctor told her to learn to live with her pain and referred her to a psychologist, who determined that her response to pain was normal. She agreed, but she wanted answers on how to take her pain away. More than anything else, she wanted to know why she was in so much pain.

If this story feels familiar to you, you are not alone. Many people with chronic pain have experienced similar frustrations. You may have even been able to relate to Sarah's feelings about her pain. Were you able to identify the characteristics of acute versus chronic pain in this story?

Let's examine chronic pain once again. Chronic pain can be present either following an injury (as in Sarah's case) or without a specific injury. For example, in disorders such as fibromyalgia (see Appendix A), individuals can experience waxing and waning symptoms of joint and muscle aches, fatigue, and insomnia. And yet there is often no specific injury to explain the original onset of pain in fibromyalgia. The diagnosis is made through excluding or eliminating specific disorders, such as rheumatoid arthritis or lupus. There is no known treatment for fibromyalgia except for addressing the insomnia and body aches. However, the experience of pain is just as complex and consuming as one stemming from a specific injury.

Whether the condition you suffer from has a clear explanation or not, the persistence of your symptoms has probably given rise to multiple consequences. In fact, the resultant feelings of isolation and despair at the loss of physical and social functioning may have become symptoms in their own right. Without effective ways of responding (called coping skills), you are likely to feel helpless and hopeless. In this program, you'll learn how to strengthen your present coping skills, as well as how to develop new ones.

Remember that your experiences are real and normal and that your responses are understandable. The fact that they are not desirable is a point in your favor. It can provide you with the perseverance to read on.

The Processes Involved in Acute and Chronic Pain

Let's take a closer look at how acute and chronic pain are created, examining each of the processes involved and the rationale for treatment.

The Role of Sensory Nerves in Pain

Under normal circumstances, nerves that carry pain messages sit quietly, waiting patiently until an event stimulates them into action. This warning system responds to events such as damaging extremes of heat and cold, trauma (either accidental or surgical), or chemical messengers (substance P, bradykinin, cytokines) released during injury or inflammation. The pain nerves carry the alarm from stimulated pain receptors located all over the body in the skin, muscles, joints, and internal organs and serve as the common pathway for pain information entering the spinal cord, no matter what the original cause of the alarm.

Among the variety of nerve fibers, there are at least two types that are thought to carry the majority of pain messages to the spinal cord: "A-delta fibers" and "C fibers." These nerves carry messages at different speeds.

A common experience may help you to understand this process. You hit the so-called funny bone in your elbow (the "funny bone" is actually your ulnar nerve). The first sensation you are likely to feel is a sharp, tingling pain. This pain sensation probably results from the activity of the A-delta nerve fibers. They carry their electrical message to the spinal cord at approximately 40 miles an hour. Usually there is a second sensation, more like an achiness, that spreads slowly up and down the inside of your arm. Such sensations are thought to result from the activity of C fibers, which carry their electrical message at approximately three miles per hour to the spinal cord. These differences in rate of speed contribute to the symphony of nerve messages involved in the pain sensation at the time of an injury. The pain pathway is a two-way street, with fast reflexes speeding from the spinal cord out to the body to put us out of harm's way (removing the hand from the hot iron) and to protect the site of injury (the spasm of surrounding muscles).

Usually when you hit your elbow, you automatically start to rub the area. This can work to soothe the painful area because other faster sensory nerve fibers, carrying pressure and touch messages to the spinal cord, are stimulated by this action. These fibers, called A-beta fibers, carry their message to the spinal cord at approximately 180 to 200 miles per hour. They race to the spinal cord to override or compete for attention with the incoming pain messages carried by the C and A-delta fibers.

Not all sensations are created equal, and you can make use of this fact for pain relief. You may have already found it helpful to apply massage, heat (including ultrasound), or ice to the painful area and/or to use transcutaneous electrical nerve stimulation (TENS) or acupuncture. These techniques can temporarily alter or decrease the pain message, depending on the intensity of the pain signal, because of the way the pain system works.

The Role of the Spinal Cord in Pain

Once a pain message has made it to the spinal cord as an electrical impulse, a very complicated system acts to send, modify, or cancel the message to the brain. Like runners in a relay race, these sensory nerves from the body hand over their pain messages to nerve cells in the spinal cord. In the spinal cord these secondary nerve cells select from the messages received based on intensity, frequency, and the overall number of competing messages from other cells connecting with them. They are influenced by excitatory chemical messages such as substance P and glutamate (targets of new pain research). They can also be influenced by inhibitory messages sent downstream from the brain. Substances such as serotonin, noradrenaline, and endorphin (*endo* = endogenous, *orphin* = morphine, the body's own natural pain reliever) are involved in pain inhibition. These inhibitory messages may alter the pain signal, allowing for changes in the intensity and meaning of the message—we call this "modulation." The modulation process helps determine just how much of the pain message gets sent to the brain to be acted on, both physically and emotionally. Thus rubbing the painful area or having a supportive spouse or friend during labor and delivery may alter the pain experience.

The Role of the Brain in Pain

Once a pain signal makes its way to the brain, the brain responds to the strength, repetition, and duration of the pain message. The brain can alter the pain message by firing impulses that make their way through the pain inhibitory system or by the release of endorphins and other "morphine-like" substances. Through connections with the cerebral cortex and limbic system (the "seat" of emotions), the pain message becomes a conscious and emotional experience. We do not see where all the electrical and chemical signals go, but we see the grimacing, limping, rubbing, and moaning that are the results of pain reaching awareness. The brain gives meaning to the pain message.

What Happens in Chronic Pain?

Chronic pain involves very complex processes in the body, at sites at which the original damage or injury occurs, as well as in the central nervous system (spinal cord and brain). These same processes are involved in acute pain. As mentioned earlier, there are diseases for which we have no cure at the moment that are associated with ongoing inflammation and tissue damage. Those diseases, such as rheumatoid arthritis, myositis, lupus, and multiple sclerosis, may be associated with chronic pain. The cause for chronic pain in these situations is thought to be related to persistent acute pain mechanisms.

Medical science has been quite ignorant of the cause of most chronic pain syndromes. Slowly, and with continuing research into the mechanisms of pain, medical scientists are discovering that certain conditions (such as an injury to a sensory nerve) may give rise to constant but previously unexplained pain. Other processes that scientists have only begun to explore, such as chronic inflammation, muscle spasms, and central nervous system mechanisms, also contribute to chronic pain.

There are diseases and therapies associated with nerve damage, such as diabetes, HIV infection, post-shingles neuropathy, and radiation/chemotherapy. We know from animal and human research that damaged pain sensory nerves can become excited all by themselves while attempting to regenerate. These normally quiet nerves can become irritable and noisy, producing spontaneous pain without any particular harmful stimulus occurring. This type of mechanism might explain some chronic pain.

Individuals who develop the pain syndrome Complex Regional Pain Syndrome Type I (once called reflex sympathetic dystrophy; see Appendix A) have pain associated with sympathetic nervous system mechanisms (such as sweating, swelling, and blood vessel constriction).

For years we have puzzled over why some people don't recover from their injuries or "successful" surgery, continuing to have pain even after the tissue has apparently healed. They may also report pain from nonpainful stimuli such as light touch or the spreading of pain beyond the original injury. Such symptoms probably reflect multiple processes. Certainly the lack of movement that commonly occurs in chronic pain weakens muscles and may cause increased discomfort in the limb that was injured. Scar tissue that develops during healing may constrict nerves and damage them.

Pain research has shown that remarkable events can occur when the spinal cord is bombarded with persistent, high levels of pain. Changes take place that magnify, spread, and perpetuate pain. These changes take place in areas of the spinal cord at which pain is modulated. They may cause the nerves to lose their ability to respond to the normal checks and balances that serve to dampen or alter the pain. Eventually the spinal cord nerves and the brain centers they serve may begin to function independently to perpetuate the pain signal long after the original injury has healed.

Why does it happen to some people and not others? Again, there are probably multiple mechanisms involved. The only consistent predictor of whether someone will develop chronic pain after an injury has been whether they reported unusually high levels of pain during the acute pain episode. Is this genetic, environmental, or a conditioned response? We don't know. Research in genetic decoding is beginning to give us tools for better identifying some of the mechanisms that may contribute to developing chronic pain, such as in certain familial migraines. But there is much to be learned.

Treating Chronic Pain

The first part of this chapter has done the following:

- Described the different parts of the normal pain pathway.
- Described the role of these parts—peripheral nerves, spinal cord, and brain—in chronic pain.
- Presented the current thinking about why chronic pain occurs.

With this groundwork laid, we look more closely at the factors that trigger or increase pain, such as inflammation, muscle spasm, nerve irritability, and mood. We look at these factors and how they influence treatment for reducing, *not curing*, chronic pain.

The Role of Inflammation in Pain

When you cut yourself, cells in the damaged area release chemicals that irritate the nerves. This causes the pain nerves to send their signal to the spinal cord, and you perceive pain, which makes you aware of the injury. Other chemicals released by damaged cells cue other responses to injury. Muscle spasms are triggered, and these protect the area from movement (see the next section). Blood vessels in the surrounding tissue constrict, allowing reduction of bleeding from the site of the injury. White blood cells and connective tissue cells start cleaning up and repairing the damage.

"Inflammation" is the body's way to fight infection or heal tissue after injury. The normal inflammation process involves cells in the body that release chemicals that then provide signals to the nerves, muscles, and blood vessels to begin the healing process. However, in chronic pain conditions such as rheumatoid arthritis, it is thought that the inflammation process has gone haywire. Instead of contributing to a normal healing process, it becomes an unregulated source of destruction.

Chronic pain syndromes associated with inflammation are lupus arthritis, ankylosing spondylitis, and possibly osteoarthritis. The extent to which inflammatory processes influence other chronic pain conditions is not known. There is a basic assumption that microinflammation may be involved in many chronic pain syndromes, and thus a trial of anti-inflammatory agents may prove beneficial.

Inflammation is treated with anti-inflammatory medications such as aspirin or ibuprofen because they block the effect of some of the chemicals that are released by the cells. Prostaglandin is one of the chemicals released during inflammation, and aspirin blocks its action. Newer anti-inflammatory agents, called COX-II inhibitors (Celebrex® and Vioxx®), may be potentially safer for long-term use. Severe inflammatory processes may also be treated with medications that block the immune system response, such as methotrexate and tumor necrosis factor inhibitors such as Embrel®, used in rheumatoid arthritis. Possible side effects of anti-inflammatory medications include the following:

- Longer bleeding times
- Stomach irritation and bleeding
- Colitis (inflammation of the colon)
- "Rebound pain"—for example, the perpetuation of headache pain as a result of continuous use of analgesic medication
- Ankle swelling
- Kidney damage

Take a moment to answer the following questions:

What anti-inflammatory medications do you use, if any? _____

_____

What is the amount per dose and how frequently do you take it? _____

_____

What possible side effects do you experience? _____

_____

The Role of Muscles in Pain

Some pain conditions are marked by their muscle spasm component. The muscles may become tight as a result of reflexive guarding of a painful area, nerve irritation, or a generalized tension response. Therefore, muscle relaxants (Norflex®, Flexeril®) are often prescribed to relax or loosen up the muscles. It is thought that these medications work primarily on the brain, except for Valium®, which also has a direct effect on skeletal muscles. (With many of these medications, it is unclear how much of the relaxation is due to the brain's relaxing and how much is due to the skeletal muscles' relaxing.) People often experience drowsiness, sedation, or impaired concentration when taking muscle relaxants because of the effect of these medications on the brain.

Other methods that are used to release muscle tension and spasm include the following:

- Muscle massage
- Acupuncture
- Application of heat or ice
- Injection of tender areas of muscle or soft tissue, called "trigger points"
- Relaxation response techniques
- Body awareness training
- Gentle stretching

The last three techniques will be addressed in detail in the next two chapters.

Take a moment to answer the following questions:

Are you taking muscle relaxants? If so, what are they? _____

_____

What is the amount per dose and how frequently do you take it? _____

_____

What possible side effects do you experience? _____

_____

What other things have you done to release muscle tension? _____

_____

Treating Pain Nerve Irritability in the Periphery and Central Nervous System

Medications may also be used to alter pain nerve irritability in the body (peripheral nerves) and in the central nervous system (spinal cord and brain). These include tricyclic antidepressants, such as amitriptyline (Elavil®), imipramine, and nortriptyline; mexiletine, an oral, Novocain®-like medicine; baclofen, used for diabetic neuropathy; Zostrix®, an ointment made from the active ingredient in red chili peppers (capsaicin); and seizure medications such as gabapentin (Neurontin®), Tegretol®, Dilantin®, and Klonopin®. A patch saturated with lidocaine (Lidoderm®) can be applied directly to the skin of those suffering from post-shingles pain. Nerve blocks with Novocain®-like substances and steroids may also be injected to quiet the firing of irritable nerves. Sumatriptan (Imitrex®) and numerous other triptan-like medications are being used for migraine headaches. Finally, direct stimulation of the peripheral nerve, spinal cord, and brain to override the pain messages from the nerves may be used to reduce chronic pain.

As research continues to help us understand what makes pain chronic, new medications and therapies will become available. In the next decade, long-acting local anesthetics may be available to block sensory nerves for months instead of minutes. Drugs aimed at disarming the mechanisms in the central nervous system that serve to wind up, magnify, and make pain persist will be developed. Ways to prevent pain from becoming chronic will be understood. It is a worldwide effort.

Take a moment to answer the following questions about your treatment:

Are you taking medications to quiet the nerve irritability? If so, what are they? _____

_____

What is the amount per dose and how frequently do you take it? _____

_____

What are the possible side effects? _____

_____

What other treatments have you tried to quiet the irritable nerves? _____

_____

Helping the Brain Help You

As mentioned before, the brain can both decrease and increase the pain experience. This modulation, like the volume control of a radio, can be influenced by a great many internal and external events.

A number of conditions impair optimum brain functioning and can actually exacerbate the pain experience; these include insomnia, depression/anxiety, and the use of alcohol. I discuss these next. The use of narcotics or opioids (e.g., morphine, hydrocodone, oxycodone, fentanyl) requires special consideration and are discussed in their own section.

Insomnia

Insomnia or poor sleep quality can make the experience of pain more difficult. Even though sleep is necessary to assure good health, just how sleep serves to rejuvenate and repair the body remains largely unknown. Many illnesses or problems, including pain, can be made worse by poor sleep.

Often patients in pain who are experiencing sleep disorders are treated with tricyclic antidepressants such as Elavil® (amitriptyline) and Desyrel® (trazodone) in low dosages to obtain a better quality of sleep. It has also been found that these medications in very low dosages appear to alter pain sensitivity in some disorders. The mechanism is unknown, but some alteration in norepinephrine and/or serotonin levels in the brain or spinal cord has been suggested. Remember that serotonin is one of the chemical messengers involved in altering or suppressing pain messages—the pain inhibitory pathways mentioned earlier. In addition, serotonin is believed to play a role in depression. This may be why antidepressants improve both depression and some chronic pain syndromes.

Other recommendations can be helpful to prepare yourself for sleep. Having a regular routine of going to bed and waking up is important. If naps are necessary, sleep only for 30–45 minutes. Taking a hot shower or bath about two hours before sleep will raise the body temperature; the cooling down afterward can help trigger sleep onset. A small carbohydrate snack before bed can induce sleep. If sleep is delayed or if you have trouble falling back to sleep for more than 30 minutes, get up and do something until you feel sleepy again. Often people become anxious as they lie in bed with their eyes wide open. Continuing to struggle with sleep simply makes it less likely to occur. The relaxation response techniques described in the next chapter will be particularly helpful when practiced before you go to bed or if you wake up during the night.

If insomnia is associated with snoring, sleep apnea (periods of not breathing while asleep), and excessive daytime drowsiness, evaluation in a sleep disorders clinic may be helpful.

Depression/Anxiety

Severe depression and anxiety disorders (such as panic attacks) can also alter the pain experience. People who experience significant depression in addition to pain have a harder time overcoming their feelings of helplessness and powerlessness. Anxious people who have pain become even more frightened by the loss of control and have a heightened level of tension. It is important to treat such disorders because of their negative influence on pain perception and self-motivation. Chapters 5 and 6 also address these feelings, as they are normally a part of many people's chronic pain experience. Disabling depression and anxiety may require medication to help bring these moods under control.

Use of Alcohol

Alcohol may temporarily alter pain perception and is an old remedy for acute pain. Alcohol does little to help with long-term coping, because nothing really changes. In those individuals who are genetically or behaviorally predisposed to it, alcoholism can be an additional complication of self-medicating pain with alcohol. In some cases, any alcohol consumption before bedtime can actually disrupt sleep. Moreover, in certain people (particularly those prone to headaches or fibromyalgia), alcohol use is associated with increased pain. As a source of empty calories with no nutritional value, alcohol can contribute to weight gain. You will have the opportunity to explore how alcohol affects your pain in Chapter 7.

Using Narcotics (Opioids) in Chronic Pain

Opioids is the more accurate name for opium-like medicines such as morphine, Percocet®, and Vicodin®. The response of chronic pain to these opioids is not the same as in acute or cancer pain. Maybe this is because the mechanisms are different, as I discussed previously. My colleagues and I do not recommend the use of opioids *in place of* taking an active role in pain management; however, opioids do have their place in helping individuals attain their goals of improved functioning. The goal of opioid treatment is not to be *pain free*, because it doesn't happen, but to have more tolerable pain. The American Pain Society and the American Academy of Pain Medicine (organizations of professional pain specialists) both endorse the careful use of opioids in chronic pain when the other treatments we have already reviewed fail to give adequate pain control. Individuals with no previous drug abuse history have few problems when one physician (usually the patient's primary care physician) prescribes a constant dose of opioids taken on a regular schedule and not erratically. Long-acting, time-release opioids are available for morphine, oxycodone, and fentanyl and tend to give a constant blood level of medication and are thought to contribute to more constant levels of pain relief. Methadone is an inexpensive, long-acting opioid alternative to the time-release opioids.

If you use a prescribed opioid, you have responsibilities. You should take the opioid only as directed, receive the opioid from one physician, and report side effects promptly, and you should not stop the drug abruptly (because of physical dependence and the possibility of withdrawal symptoms). You should also use caution in the first few weeks of dose adjustments, as impairment in thinking, judgment, and reaction time may occur at that time. When using an opioid you are also expected to use other pain management skills such as described in this book to reduce the amount of opioid needed. For example, with such skills you can attend to the other symptoms associated with chronic pain, such as insomnia, anxiety, muscle tension, and fatigue. Often opioids are misused in chronic pain because people lack the skills to cope with pain in any other way. Problems may develop when pain medications are taken to "relax," to induce sleep, to decrease the fear of anticipated pain increases, to reduce stress-based symptoms, or to alleviate frustration. These purposes are better served by using techniques such as those described in this book.

It is important that you discuss any side effects (nausea, constipation, drowsiness) of opioid treatment with your health care professional. These can be treated effectively and should be if the opioid is making a significant difference in pain control. The goal of opioid therapy is better pain control in order to allow more activities to occur. What activities are being stopped by your high pain level? Make a list. For example, exercise, shopping, sitting at the computer, going to the theater, or volunteering. Of course, important pacing and realistic goal setting (covered in the upcoming chapters) will help you be more successful.

It should be noted that if you do take opioids on a daily basis that you will most likely need additional opioids for post-surgical pain control. After surgery you will need your daily dose of opioids plus up to two to three times more than an individual would require who was not taking chronic opioids before surgery. Many doctors and nurses are not aware of this so it is important for you to discuss the post-operative pain treatment before surgery if possible with the anesthesiologist or surgeon who will be working with you. Likewise, should you incur a new painful injury, such as a bone fracture or passing kidney stones, you will also need additional opioids added to your regimen. These increases in opioids should not be required for more than the average recovery period.

There are patients whose pain does not respond to opioids. They find that the pain does not really change that much on or off the medication. They may even feel better once the opioid is tapered and stopped. The long-term effects of opioid treatment for chronic pain are not known. In spite of this, some patients are definitely benefited, and opioids should be considered on a case-by-case basis. Consultation with a pain specialist may provide guidance on how to proceed.

The Good News

Just as insomnia, depression/anxiety, and use of alcohol can impair optimum brain functioning and make your pain experience worse, there are ways of altering brain activity that can change your pain experience in positive, healthy ways. These include consciously distracting yourself; increasing endorphins, the natural brain "narcotics"; or engaging in pleasurable activities, relaxation techniques, exercise, and/or stress management. These techniques are presented in detail in the chapters to follow.

Take a moment to answer the following questions:

Are you taking antidepressants for depression and/or anxiety? If so, what are they? _____

_____

What is the amount per dose and how frequently do you take it? _____

_____

What are the possible side effects? _____

_____

Are you taking opioids? If so, what are they? _____

_____

What is the amount per dose and how frequently do you take it? _____

_____

What possible side effects do you experience? _____

_____

What side effect treatments do you use? _____

_____

Are you using any other medications for pain management that we haven't mentioned? If so what are they? _____

_____

Do you understand why these medication(s) have been recommended? If not, whom can you ask for information? _____

Despite what we do know about pain, the fact remains that we are not able to take away chronic pain for the millions who suffer with it, but the suffering is optional.

The Meanings of Pain

Cultural Influences on Attitudes toward Pain

The way pain is treated in the Western hemisphere is strongly influenced by Western culture. The presence of a booming pharmacological industry has created a subtle but highly influential attitude toward pain treatment. The emphasis is on "quick fixes" and medications for all our problems. There is much less emphasis on what patients can do for themselves to make their lives healthier and happier. Medicine does not have all the answers yet. The erroneous impression that it does is pervasive. David Morris comments on this in his book *The Culture of Pain*:

> Today our culture has willingly, almost gratefully, handed over to medicine the job of explaining pain. This development, accelerating with the prestige of science over the last several centuries, has brought with it consequences that remain almost completely unanalyzed. . . . Although almost all eras and cultures have employed doctors, never before in human history has the explanation of pain fallen so completely to medicine. (p. 19)

With the current incomplete state of medical knowledge, solutions shouldn't be limited to drugs or medical procedures. Yet many patients are unaware that "medicine knows all" is only a cultural expectation, not a fact. They have not had the opportunity to explore the various influences on their pain experiences. This program will help you explore the multiple meanings of pain and will help you see that different attitudes toward pain are possible.

Exercise: Exploring the Meanings of Pain

Let's begin with an exercise that helps you explore how your pain has affected your activities, physical responses, thoughts, and feelings. Don't be surprised or alarmed if your responses to these questions cause you sadness, anger, or anxiety. This exercise will help you start to assess the full cost of your pain experience. It will also help you to begin to recognize any ineffective coping processes, so that you can replace them with more effective ones in the chapters to come.

1. How has your pain affected how you work, play, and perform other activities?

    _____

    _____

    _____

    _____

    _____

    _____

2. What other physical symptoms do you experience in addition to the pain (for example, insomnia, fatigue, etc.)? _____

    _____

    _____

    _____

    _____

    _____

3. What are your thoughts and feelings in response to your pain experience? _____

_____

_____

_____

_____

_____

_____

4. What does being in pain mean to you?

_____

_____

_____

_____

_____

_____

Please do the above exercise before continuing. It will help you understand what follows.

When I have patients do this exercise in the clinical programs I conduct, the blackboard is filled with the real consequences of their daily pain. Samples of some of these responses are given in the table below. It is clear just how courageous these people have been to continue with their lives in spite of their suffering. For most, all aspects of their lives have been affected, and though it has been difficult they have done the best they can. What becomes striking during the discussion that follows the exercise, however, is that for most of these people only their *physical* pain has been the focus of their medical treatment. The emotional, thinking, and behavioral components of their pain experience have been ignored.

Activities decreased or stopped	Physical symptoms	Feelings and thoughts
Work	Fatigue	Anger
Pleasure (hobbies, movies)	Sweating	Depression
Household chores	Weight gain/loss	Anxiety
Sex	Headaches	Fear
Socializing	Decreased concentration	Guilt
Exercise	Palpitations (increased heart rate)	Frustration
Family activities	Shortness of breath	Out of control
Sports	Decreased memory	Can't do what I used to
	Diarrhea	Hopeless/helpless

(cont.)

Activities decreased or stopped	Physical symptoms	Feelings and thoughts
Sports *(cont.)*	Headaches	No one understands
	Muscle tension	"Why me?"
	Insomnia	"When will this go away?"
	Constipation	"I can't go on."
	Body aches	Failure
		Unlovable
		Ugly
		Denial

The Division of Mind and Body

Much of the suffering you have identified in the previous exercise arises out of a common misunderstanding in Western culture that there is a division between mind and body. This division is reinforced daily. Medical doctors take care of our bodies, and psychologists or psychiatrists take care of our minds. Our hearts are looked after by heart specialists, our stomachs by stomach specialists, and so on. In the last 20 years there has been a growing discontent with the fragmentation of our bodies and minds. Such terms as "behavioral medicine" and "holistic medicine" have been used to describe the integration of mind and body in medical practice. Now with the emphasis on managed care and universal health coverage, there is a growing awareness that if the fragmentation of people's health care does not provide enough impetus for change, the outrageous costs generated by such fragmentation certainly do.

The division of mind and body is a false one, and nowhere is it more ineffective than in dealing with chronic pain. The experience of pain is a coming together of multiple factors, such as the following:

- The pain signal
- Expectations of yourself and of others
- Self-esteem
- Ability to function
- Temperature variations
- Hormones
- Genetics
- Previous traumas
- Injustices and beliefs

To deny these influences or to act as if nothing is wrong is not in your best interests, nor is it effective in terms of coping. If you deny the pain and push on, or regularly engage in activities that increase the pain, you only increase the severity of your condition. Even if the consequences aren't immediate (you can't get out of bed), they are cumulative (stress symptoms). As a result, you are setting yourself up for endless frustration and loss of control.

However, pretending that nothing is wrong is not to be confused with making a conscious decision to increase activity for a particular purpose in the knowledge that increased discomfort will follow. For example, Mary wanted to take her granddaughter to the circus. She knew that sitting through the performance would increase her pain. She prepared herself with an extra cushion and sat in the back row so that she could stand periodically. Her pain did increase, but she was not upset because she had felt it to be worth the effort, and her granddaughter was thrilled. The decision was her choice and was under her control.

The key here is to ask, "Where do I have control?" If you can acknowledge your pain and make conscious decisions about your activities, you will not feel so victimized. As one patient said, "If I sit, I'm in pain. If I walk, I'm in pain. So I might as well walk and get somewhere." If the pain is part of your life, it is important to work with it; this is where you have the control.

You probably feel a fair amount of external pressure to act as if nothing is wrong and to ignore what you know to be necessary. You can change your attitude toward your pain, increase your activities safely, and have a life in addition to the pain. The rest of this book will help you do just that.

The misunderstandings that arise out of the separation of mind and body are not limited to people who actually experience chronic pain. The refusal of many physicians to acknowledge that physical pain is associated with psychological suffering gives rise to the "psychological illness" stigma. When people express sadness or anxiety about their pain, it is often assumed that these emotional symptoms are the *cause* of their pain. There is a tendency to label such people as "hysterics" or "hypochondriacs" or to dismiss the problem as "not real" (i.e., not physical). Many individuals experience this stigma when their physicians cannot explain the physical cause of persistent pain.

Likewise, the failure to address psychological and sociological issues early in the course of pain management devalues these important aspects of the pain experience. Such skills as relaxation techniques are usually offered only *after* a patient has "failed" to respond to medications or nerve blocks. Until recently, primary care physicians received no formal training in forms of pain management other than the use of medications. And pain management is still included in only a minority of physician training programs. Mind–body approaches to pain management have been overlooked not because they are ineffective but simply because they remain unknown to those providing the majority of the therapy.

So what is the problem? And whose problem is it, anyway? The problem is, of course, that you have pain, and it is not going away. And, in keeping with the philosophy of this program, I strongly recommend that you acknowledge the problem is yours, since you are the one in pain. If you hand it over to your physician, family, or society, you simply perpetuate your loss of control.

Where Do You Go from Here?

In the following chapters, the physical symptoms that you have identified in the previous exercise are addressed through a series of skills and techniques aimed at reducing stress. These symptoms are manifestations of the wear and tear on the body resulting from prolonged pain and the failure to heed the mind–body, body–mind connection. Such techniques as the relaxation response, breath exercises, stretching, and body awareness exercises will help you nurture your body and counteract the stress symptoms.

The decreases you have identified in your physical activities and socialization, along with increased isolation, will be addressed in various ways. You will learn to monitor the way you pace yourself in performing activities, to interpret your pain sensations, and to add pleasurable activities and exercise to your regular routine.

The negative or self-defeating thoughts and feelings you have identified will be approached through cognitive therapy techniques. These include the identification of negative self-talk, fed by assumptions of how things should proceed in life and distortions of what is really happening around you. You will learn how to be more realistic and self-empowering. Humor will be used to soften the hard work and slow pace at which real change proceeds. Communication skills will encourage self-esteem and the assertiveness required to identify your needs. Improving your problem-solving abilities in regard to the challenges of pain will allow you to participate fully in society once again and to achieve the goals you set for yourself.

Summary

Pain

- Pain is a symptom that indicates harm to the body.
- People's perceptions can alter their pain experience in various ways.
- There are two categories of pain:

  - Acute pain is limited in duration, and the cause is usually known.
  - Chronic pain lasts longer than three months, and is the result of multiple mechanisms, most of which are not fully understood.

Nerves

- There are two types of sensory nerve fibers that carry the pain message to the spinal cord:

  - A-delta fibers carry the message to the spinal cord at approximately 40 miles per hour.
  - C fibers carry the message to the spinal cord at approximately 3 miles per hour.

- Pain nerves are stimulated by extremes of hot or cold, trauma, or chemicals released during inflammation.
- Not all nerves carry the same message, and not all pain messages are paid attention to.
- There is competition among the messages as they come into the spinal cord; as a result, some pain can be reduced by rubbing, by applying pressure, or by other means.
- Chronic pain is probably the result of the pain system losing the normal checks and balances involved in modulating pain signals.
- Chronic pain may also develop when an injured pain nerve attempts to regenerate.
- Sometimes medications are effective in calming the irritated nerves.

Inflammation

- Inflammation is a process that fights infection or cleans up and repairs tissue damage.
- When inflammation occurs, cells in the body release chemicals as a signal to the nerves, muscles, and blood vessels that damage control must begin.
- Inflammation is treated with anti-inflammatory medications such as aspirin or ibuprofen, because they block the effects of some of the chemicals that are released.

Muscles

- Muscle spasm or tightness can be the result of a guarding of the painful area, nerve irritation, or a generalized tension response.
- Muscle relaxants are thought to work primarily in the brain to loosen up the muscles.
- Other ways to release muscle tension and spasm include massage, acupuncture, heat/ice application, trigger point injections, relaxation response techniques, and body awareness training.

Central Nervous System

- Pain signals carried by the nerves arrive in the spinal cord as electrical impulses.
- These electrical impulses connect with specific areas that send the stimulus to another level of the spinal cord, to the brain, or to both areas.
- The nerve signals may also be modulated through inhibitory pathways from the brain, which can alter the pain signals.
- The brain gives meaning to the pain message.
- If brain function is impaired or if the brain is distracted, the pain experience is altered.
- Sleep disorders can make the pain experience more difficult. Tricyclic antidepres-

sants are used to treat sleep disorders and ease the pain experience; these antidepressants in low dosages also appear to alter pain sensitivity.

- Severe depression and anxiety disorders can exacerbate the pain experience.
- The use of opioids should be decided on an individual basis with the treating physician.
- The goal of opioid treatment in chronic pain is to reduce disabling pain and increase activities.
- There are guidelines for using opioids in chronic pain.
- The use of alcohol does little to help with long-term coping, carries the risk of abuse, and can actually disrupt sleep and increase pain.

The Meanings of Pain

- The idea that medicine has all the answers for pain is pervasive in Western culture.
- Chronic pain has multiple meanings for everyone who suffers from it.
- The experience of pain involves both mind *and* body; many patients have suffered from the artificial division between mind and body.
- Physical pain is associated with psychological suffering.
- By acknowledging the pain and making conscious decisions about your activities, you will gain some control over it.

Exploration Tasks

1. Answer all the questions in this chapter on medication, and get information from your pharmacist or the *Physicians' Desk Reference* on each medication that you take.
2. Make up an index card with all your medications and doses and how often you take them. Carry this card in your purse or wallet.

Supplementary Reading

The following books provide additional information on the pain process and on maintaining health:

Herbert Benson and Eileen Stuart, *The Wellness Book: The Comprehensive Guide to Maintaining Health and Treating Stress-Related Illness* (New York: Fireside, 1993).

Howard L. Fields, *Pain Mechanisms and Management, Second Edition* (New York: McGraw-Hill, 2001).

David Morris, *The Culture of Pain* (Berkeley: University of California Press, 1991).

Robert Ornstein and David Sobel, *The Healing Brain* (Los Altos, CA: Malor Books, 1999).

Patrick Wall and Steven Rose (Eds.), *Pain: The Science of Suffering* (New York: Columbia University Press, 2000).

Chapter 3

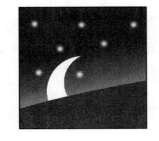

The Mind–Body Connection

> I had forgotten that my body was also a sanctuary, a haven. . . . I felt it had betrayed me and tortured me for so many years.

The above comment was made by Mary, a program participant, about her pain experience after practicing the techniques that are described in this chapter.

Chronic Pain as a Form of Chronic Stress

As indicated in Chapter 2, the mind and body are really one. They never have been separate and never should have been viewed as separate. How you feel (happy, sad, angry) can influence and be influenced by your body's processes. For instance, you may have noticed that on a day when your pain is particularly bad, you have trouble concentrating or lose your appetite. You may have also noticed that when you are intensely focused on an activity (such as watching a football playoff or talking with your best friend), your pain, for that time, slips out of consciousness. Because this mind–body connection is so intimate, the experience of "stress"—defined here as the *perception* of a physical or psychological threat and the *perception* of being ill prepared to cope with the threat—can be associated with both physical and emotional symptoms.

Human beings are biologically prepared with an automatic response to the perception of threat or danger, called the "fight-or-flight response." It is caused by the release of adrenalin from the sympathetic nervous system and other hormones, such as cortisol and growth hormone. Let's look at the following scenario:

It is late at night and you are home alone. You wake up to the sound of a crash downstairs. Your heart starts to beat rapidly; your muscles tense up; you feel anxious and short of breath. You may not be aware of it, but the hair on the back of your neck is standing on end, and your blood pressure is increasing. Blood is moving from your stomach to your skeletal muscles. Your body is preparing to fight or flee.

The first thing you do is grab a candlestick and quietly make your way downstairs. Trembling, you listen for further sounds. As you reach the bottom of the stairs, you see that the "intruder" is your cat dashing away from a broken vase. Within minutes after the "danger" has passed, your physical symptoms return to normal and your fear passes.

The changes in your body that constitute the fight-or-flight response (increased heart and breath rate, increased blood pressure, changing of blood flow to muscles, etc.) are meant to be a temporary overdrive system for meeting the challenge of threat or danger. When you are in a perpetually stressed state, however, your body can be extended beyond its capacity for reestablishing homeostasis (balance). Your recuperative abilities can be exhausted. This can contribute to numerous symptoms:

- Reduced immunity to disease
- Diarrhea and/or constipation
- Sleep disturbance
- Fatigue
- Headaches
- Poor concentration
- Shortness of breath
- Weight loss/gain
- Increased muscle tension
- Anxiety/depression

Chronic pain certainly fits the definition of adverse chronic stress. The effects of chronic stress are felt to be the results of a prolonged fight-or-flight response. In addition to the physical stress chronic pain places on your body, your experience of pain can be increased or decreased by how you perceive your ability to cope with the pain. (This is true of other stressors as well.) If you feel overwhelmed as a result of your pain and do not take time to balance the stress effects of the pain, you will most likely begin to experience other stress-related symptoms such as those listed here. This is why stress management techniques can be so helpful in coping with chronic pain.

Techniques that bring about the "relaxation response," as described next, will help you alter the physical symptoms of stress; they will also prepare you to cope more effectively with the stress of pain.

The Relaxation Response (RR) Is Not the Same as Relaxing

The "relaxation response" (which will be abbreviated from here on in this book as "RR") was first described by Herbert Benson and his colleagues at Harvard Medical School in the early 1970s. In contrast to the fight-or-flight response, the RR appears to play a role in quieting the body's responses to stress. However, unlike the fight-or-flight response, the RR is not automatic. Development of the RR requires practice with certain mental techniques before it can be called on to counteract stress.

After reviewing many religious and philosophical writings, Benson realized that for centuries humankind had been provided with instructions for bringing about this quieting reflex. He also *realized* that even though many techniques could bring about this natural bodily response, there were two simple steps common to them all:

1. Focusing one's mind on a repetitive phrase, word, breath, or action.
2. Adopting a passive attitude toward the thoughts that go through one's head.

We know through extensive research done by Benson and others that the regular practice of techniques that bring about the RR is associated with a general decrease in responsiveness to the arousal of the sympathetic nervous system. Hence, those symptoms that are the results of chronic stress are particularly affected. The physical effects of the RR can be divided into (1) immediate changes, which occur while a person is focusing on a repetitive word, phrase, breath, or action; and (2) long-term changes, which occur after repeated practice for at least a month and are present even when a person is not sitting quietly practicing an RR technique. The more immediate changes include a lowering of blood pressure, heart rate, breath rate, and oxygen consumption (which is a measure of metabolic rate). The long-term changes are thought to alter the body's response to adrenalin. People may report a decrease in anxiety and depression, as well as an improvement in their ability to cope with life stressors, after regular practice of their RR techniques.

Many people confuse "feeling relaxed" with the RR. They are not the same unless what a person is doing to relax includes the two steps mentioned—focus on a repetitive stimulus and passive attitude. In research using the RR, the controls—that is, the participants who will *not* be taught how to bring about the RR—are instructed instead to listen to music or read a book. Although under normal circumstances listening to music and reading a book may be relaxing, they do not bring about the RR.

In summary, the RR is a natural response of the body, but it needs to be trained and practiced. It is brought about through a focusing of the mind on a repetitive word, phrase, breath, or action, and through passive regard to interfering thoughts. It is not elicited by reading a book, listening to quiet music, sleeping, or hanging out. All of these may be relaxing, but they are not the same as bringing about the RR.

Using Breath to Relax and Focus Your Mind

The key to bringing about the RR is focused awareness. Your breathing can be the object of that focus. In addition, because the normal breathing patterns can be disrupted by tension, stress, and pain, focusing on how you breathe may provide you with an additional method of relaxing.

There are two types of breathing: "chest breathing" and "diaphragmatic breathing" (better known as "abdominal breathing").

Chest Breathing

Many people, particularly women, are "chest breathers." That is, they suck in their abdomens and expand their chests with each in-breath. In Western culture, women are taught early in life that the "proper" posture is one in which the abdomen is flat at all times. This posture is difficult to maintain if a person breathes from the abdomen or "diaphragmatically," which requires the stomach to move in and out with each breath.

Many men and women also become chest breathers because of prolonged anxiety, stress, and tension. One reason for this may be that short, shallow breaths are characteristic of anxiety. Stress may also increase tension in the abdominal area, not allowing the diaphragm to contract completely or the abdominal wall to move out when taking an in-breath. Only the chest expands as a result, and the breath is not as deep.

Diaphragmatic Breathing

We all start out breathing diaphragmatically, with our abdomens rising and falling. Watch infants when they breathe: Their stomachs move with each breath. Over the years, many of us become chest breathers. Relearning to breathe diaphragmatically may feel strange at first, but with practice it can become second nature again.

The diaphragm is a thin dome of muscle that separates the chest cavity from the abdominal cavity. At the beginning of each in-breath, it contracts and the dome flattens out. Air is then pulled into the lungs, and the abdominal wall moves out. (Picture a balloon in the abdomen that fills with air on the in-breath.) When the diaphragm and the chest relax, the breath moves out and the abdomen flattens again. On the next in-breath, the process starts over. Because of this extra space for the lungs to fill, a diaphragmatic breath is a fuller and more complete breath than a chest breath.

For reasons that are still not altogether clear to physiologists, diaphragmatic breathing can bring about a feeling of calm and relaxation when it is purposefully done.

Breathing Exercises

It is recommended that you wear loose, comfortable clothing and that you find a quiet, relaxing place to engage in breathing exercises.

How Do You Breathe?

Before starting these exercises, you need to become aware of how you breathe.

1. Find a comfortable place and lie down on your back. If this is uncomfortable, try sitting in a chair.
2. Place one hand on your breastbone and one hand over your belly button.
3. Close your eyes and become aware of what is moving when you breathe in and out.
4. If your abdomen moves up and down (without your forcing it) with each breath, you are already breathing diaphragmatically. You can move on to the "Breath-Focusing Exercises" section later in this chapter. If your chest moves up and down with each breath, however, you need to practice breathing diaphragmatically. Go to the next section, "Diaphragmatic Breathing Exercises."

Diaphragmatic Breathing Exercises

Three diaphragmatic breathing exercises are provided here to help you train your awareness of what should be moving when you breathe diaphragmatically. If one position does not work out for you, try another. Once you are aware, you should be able to do diaphragmatic or abdominal breathing lying, sitting, or standing.

Sometimes when people focus on their breath, they tend to breathe too fast or too deeply. If you feel light-headed, dizzy, or anxious, you may be breathing too quickly or too deeply; just stop practicing for a moment and breathe normally until the symptoms pass. In addition, *do not do these exercises if these positions make your pain worse.*

Exercise 1

1. Find a comfortable place and lie on your stomach.
2. Lift your chest off the floor by bringing your elbows back against your side at the level of your shoulders. Then push off the floor with your forearms (like the Sphinx). This position will arch your back slightly.
3. Breathe normally. This will lock your chest so that when you breathe, the abdomen alone will move up and down.

Exercise 2

1. Sit in a chair and clasp your hands behind your head.
2. Point your elbows out to the side. Again, this serves to lock your chest so that you can feel the movement in your abdomen.
3. Breathe normally.

Exercise 3

1. Find a comfortable place and lie on your back.
2. Place your hands just below your belly button.
3. Close your eyes and imagine a balloon inside your abdomen.
4. Each time you breathe in, imagine the balloon filling with air.
5. Each time you breathe out, imagine the balloon collapsing.

Breath-Focusing Exercises

Now that you are aware of your breathing, you can start to practice breath focusing.

1. Make a tight fist and notice what happens to your breathing. Don't read on; just do it. Did you find that you held your breath or breathed in shallow, short spurts?
2. Now relax that fist.
3. Make a tight fist again, but this time continue to breathe normally. What happens to the tension in your fist? The tension should be reduced—and, in fact, should be difficult to maintain without a real effort.

Remember: *It's hard to maintain tension (stress, pain, anger, anxiety) and keep breathing.* This principle is used in Lamaze exercises for women in labor. The Lamaze technique focuses on breathing to release tension and increase control during the various stages of labor. Women are encouraged to use their breathing to control the pain. This same principle can be applied to your pain experience.

Observe how often you hold your breath when you anticipate pain or when you are experiencing pain. You can change this experience by breathing. When you experience pain (or increased tension, anger, anxiety, or stress), do the following:

1. Purposefully stop and pause.
2. Take a slow, deep breath from your diaphragm.
3. Focus on what you are doing and how you are feeling. What is the problem? What are your choices? Do you need to continue with a certain activity, or can you change what you are doing? Is the situation worth getting upset about at this moment?

As you will see, breath-focusing exercises can sometimes give you instant control, because they make you focus on the present moment. You may often be caught off guard by stressful events if you are busy worrying about the future, wishing you could change the past, or responding automatically without thinking at all. Focusing on the present moment allows you to consider more clearly what has gotten you upset. Many times, all you need to do is to make a change in the way you are doing or thinking about something.

Focusing on your breath and breathing diaphragmatically can also get you through uncomfortable or difficult procedures such as magnetic resonance imaging (MRI), pelvic exams, sigmoidoscopies, and injections. In fact, many of life's challenges can be made a little easier by just breathing. Make breath-focusing exercises a part of your daily routine.

Mini-Relaxations

When you take a moment and focus on diaphragmatic breathing, think of this as a "mini-relaxation." Begin to practice mini-relaxations during the day to release tension that has accumulated over short periods of time. Here are some suggestions for different kinds of mini-relaxations:

1. Whenever you have just a minute, take a deep breath; as you breathe out, imagine all the tension in your body and mind leaving through this breath.
2. Take a moment to tense all the muscles you can at once. Then take a deep breath and slowly breathe out, letting all the tension go. Repeat this mini-relaxation until you have reduced the tension.
3. Take an inventory of body tension in your familiar stress points. For example, is there tension in your neck or upper back? If you find that there is, pretend that you can direct the breath into that area of tension. As you breathe out, feel the tension release.
4. Count to 10 taking a slow, deep breath. Hold the breath for one count. Then breathe out slowly, again as you count to 10.

Preparing to Practice Eliciting the RR

Minimizing Distractions and Making Yourself Comfortable

To minimize distractions, find a quiet, comfortable place where you feel safe practicing the RR techniques to be described later. If necessary, put a "Do Not Disturb" sign (provided at the end of this book) on the door and take the phone off the hook.

By all means, respect your needs for comfort and find the position that feels best to you. The following are suggestions for making yourself comfortable:

1. Use a heating pad, ice, and/or supportive pillows to make yourself as comfortable as needed.
2. Make sure the temperature in the room is right for you, or have a blanket nearby if you should become chilled.
3. If you prefer to lie down while eliciting the RR, but find yourself falling asleep, try a sitting position. A good compromise between lying down and sitting is using a reclining chair.
4. Pick a time to do your RR practice when your pain is not at its worst.
5. Practice an RR technique for 20 minutes once a day, or for 10 minutes twice a day.

6. When you end your session, always count to three and slowly open your eyes. Get up slowly, so that your body will adjust to the postural change after such deep relaxation.

7. Do not set an alarm. If you are not using a relaxation tape and want to keep track of the time, just set a clock in front of you and open your eyes periodically. After practicing a few times, you will usually be able to judge when 20 minutes have elapsed.

Using Relaxation Tapes

Relaxation tapes can be quite valuable when you are first learning an RR technique. These tapes can often be found in health food stores and "New Age" shops. Tapes of environmental sounds and music for meditation are also available in many stores. The Mind/Body Medical Institute, under the direction of Herbert Benson at the Beth Israel Deaconess Medical Center in Boston, has a wide variety of relaxation tapes from which to choose. The tapes we used in the pain program at the Beth Israel Deaconess Medical Center are also available; call (617) 632-9530 for information.

My colleagues and I recommend that in the beginning you keep to a simple technique (see "Basic RR Techniques," later in this chapter). Also, changing tapes or focus word(s) every other day will not help you focus your mind. Consistency is important. Use a tape (or word, phrase, or breath) for some time before deciding that you need to make a change.

Mind Chatter

At times your thoughts may feel as if they are going in many different directions at once, and the resulting chatter of your mind may sound like a cast of thousands. This can be very distracting as it seems to go on and on, and it can affect your concentration. It happens to all of us; it shows us that we can sometimes be someplace mentally and another place physically. For instance, you may be thinking about something that happened in the past, or you may be planning for the future. It's difficult not to get caught up in these random thoughts.

There is a time and place for this "mind chatter," but it always seems to get louder when you are trying to practice an RR technique. Mind chatter is persistent, and you may find that it creeps into your consciousness even as you assume a passive attitude. Use your breathing or your focus word or phrase (see RR Technique 1, in the next section) to reduce or even temporarily eliminate the mind chatter.

Problem Solving

The intent of this section is to help you overcome any obstacles that may prevent you from practicing the RR techniques. No doubt you could always find a hundred reasons not to do your RR practice, so this section could also be called "No Excuses!"

The following are the most commonly expressed problems that participants experience in this program. After reading this section, you should feel better about how you handle any obstacles that prevent you from practicing the RR techniques.

Lack of Time

"I don't have the time!" you may exclaim. The response to this is simple: If you want to feel better, *make* the time. First, ask yourself why you feel you don't have the time. Do these answers from previous program participants seem familiar?

> "What will people think if they see me doing nothing? I do so little as it is."

> "My family needs me."

> "This can't possibly make a difference—my pain is real."

> "I'm in too much pain."

Such statements may result from an attitude that gives too much control to others; from low self-esteem or learned helplessness; or simply from practicing at times when your pain is the worst or you're too exhausted. These are all normal feelings, but you won't feel any better unless you overcome them and adopt an attitude that involves doing what is recommended. Your choice is "to do or not to do." When you choose "to do," you have the opportunity to experience all the positive benefits of bringing about the RR and reducing your stress.

Increased Awareness of Pain

You may find, as have many other people, that you experience an increased awareness of your pain when you have minimized external distractions and attempt to practice an RR technique. Sometimes when you close your eyes in a quiet room, the pain comes roaring back.

Try finding a comfortable position when your pain is at its least. If this fails, practice RR Technique 6 (self-hypnosis), described later in this chapter. Sometimes just focusing all of your attention on the pain will at first increase it, but within seconds this awareness should diminish. As indicated in Chapter 2, the brain is not "wired" to pay attention to constant or unvaried stimulation.

A meditation technique called "mindfulness" is described by Jon Kabat-Zinn in his book *Full Catastrophe Living* (see "Supplementary Reading" at the end of this chapter). This technique encourages you to let the mind stay passively focused on the pain. Allow yourself simply to *observe* the pain and the feelings you may have, such as fear or anger, without running away from those feelings or the sensation. And say to yourself, "Oh, yes, that's my pain and that's my anger." This technique can have dramatic results, because by staying focused on the pain you begin to realize how much fighting your pain or avoiding those feelings contribute to your feeling powerless. Once you understand this, then, every time the pain tugs at your awareness, you do not have to let it control you by feeding it with anger, anxiety, or frustration. Now return to your focus word, phrase, or breath. This may seem impossible to do. You may want to ignore your pain, because you may fear that your pain will get worse. It will not. This is a very powerful way of identifying the fact that the pain exists and that you are the one who experiences the pain. How you choose to feel about your pain is under your control.

Problems with Sitting Still or Relaxing

You may say, "I can't sit still. I'm not the kind of person to relax; I must be busy. I feel anxious when I start to relax or close my eyes." If this is so, ask yourself why you can't sit still.

To begin with, do you like your own company? Do you only feel worthwhile if you're doing something? Some people have such a fragile sense of self-worth and self-esteem that they are the last people they want to sit or be alone with. In fact, they don't like their own company. Others feel that meeting others' demands is the only activity that counts. This makes sitting quietly and bringing about the RR seem like an "irresponsible" thing to do. Still others may be so physically tense that they don't know what it's like to relax (in mind or body!).

If you are physically tense, some gentle stretching or the systematic contracting and relaxing of various muscle groups, as in "progressive muscle relaxation" (see RR Technique 3 in the next section), may be helpful. If your self-esteem is vulnerable and/or your need to meet others' demands is high, you may find the following recommendation helpful. At the beginning of your RR practice, take a moment to imagine a covered basket or toolbox sitting beside you. Identify the thoughts that are going through your head that are causing worry or concerns. As you identify these items you imagine opening the basket or toolbox cover and depositing the items. Make an agreement with yourself that you can take all those things out right after you do your RR session but that, while you are engaged in the RR practice, they are to remain inside the container where you've placed them. It is surprising how effective this simple negotiation with yourself can be when *you* decide when you will or won't be distracted or worried.

There are some people who have trouble relaxing because they are trying to avoid memories of traumatic events, such as physical or sexual abuse. This inability to relax is associated with hypervigilance (being on guard against harm) and has been described in various posttraumatic stress syndromes. For some, these traumatic memories surface whenever they let their guard down and relax. For others, these memories have been hidden from consciousness until they started to practice the RR techniques.

My colleagues and I have found that these memories needn't deter someone from enjoying the benefits of the RR. There are ways of modifying the RR techniques to minimize the anxiety. Furthermore, because these feelings of past trauma tend to magnify the negative feelings of vulnerability, being out of control, and "no one believes me" that are characteristic of chronic pain, it is important that the two experiences—previous trauma and present chronic pain—be differentiated.

It is not possible to give universal recommendations for some very complicated reactions to trauma. The following, however, are suggestions to help decrease the discomfort of these feelings.

1. Acknowledge that you are indeed a very special person for having taken the initiative to pick up this book. Parts of you sense that the way things have been going are not good and that there must be a better way. Hang on to this self-awareness; it can get you through the rough times. Change is not easy and rarely proceeds without effort.

2. Practice your RR techniques in a safe place, with locked doors and the lights on if necessary. Do whatever it takes to make yourself feel comfortable. Sometimes if you create a safe physical environment, a safe internal state can follow.

3. Use a relaxation tape to minimize internal distractions. Keep your eyes open or stare at a candle flame as a focus. Do progressive muscle relaxation or engage in an exercise in which you can couple movement and breath focus. This, too, will help cut down on the internal distractions.

4. Biofeedback therapy can sometimes be very helpful, because it allows for external feedback of internal processes—such as muscle tension, skin conductance, or skin temperature—while you are learning to relax. Biofeedback devices keep your attention focused on changing these physical parameters until you are comfortable enough to do so on your own without the machine.

5. Psychotherapy with someone familiar with the problems of various posttraumatic stress syndromes can also support your efforts. In our experience, once the memories are identified, they will not be suppressed out of consciousness again. However, their conscious presence may indicate that you are now ready to deal with the memories. If possible, try to come to terms with your past experiences and memories, because they do have an impact on your pain experience and can be serious stressors in their own right. *Seek help and take care of yourself.*

Peculiar Sensations or Experiences

Although it is a rare complaint, some program participants have reported out-of-body experiences, dissociation, or feelings of a presence other than their own. In most of these cases, the persons have been practicing an RR technique for longer than recommended—more than one hour, or several times a day for an hour or more. This is an instance in which doing something more, or more often, is not necessarily better for you. Overuse of such techniques can lead to alterations in consciousness, and it is therefore important to follow the specific instructions. The techniques presented in the next session are safe and very effective if used as instructed.

Some people are so used to feeling "wired" that feeling relaxed feels peculiar to them. If this is the case *for* you, you may just need to learn what it feels like to be relaxed.

Seizure Disorders

If you have a seizure disorder, it is suggested that you practice your RR techniques while lying down. Some seizures are brought on by a change in level of arousal, such as going to sleep or awakening. Because the brain waves associated with bringing about the RR are identical to those occurring in the first stage of sleep, people with sleep-onset seizure disorders may experience their seizures when they first start practicing. This may pass with continued practice or with the use of another technique (progressive muscle relaxation, yoga, or another physically focused repetitive technique). Other people have found that they can actually *control* their seizures by practicing the RR techniques, learning to relax, and redirecting their focus of attention at the onset of the warning signal that sometimes occurs before a seizure.

Insulin-Dependent Diabetes

Adrenalin can alter insulin availability, making it necessary for more insulin to be in circulation to produce the same sugar-lowering effect; therefore, stress can increase insulin requirements. Many patients on insulin find that their insulin requirement is reduced after starting regular practice of an RR technique. If you are an insulin-dependent diabetic, take hypoglycemic reactions *seriously* and reduce your insulin intake if you begin to experience lower blood sugar levels.

Hypertension

Antihypertensive medications can interfere with the normal adjustments to postural changes. If you have hypertension, make sure you change positions (from lying to sitting or from sitting to standing) *slowly* after your RR practice. Many patients find that with regular practice of RR techniques, their blood pressure may decrease, and their medication requirements may even be reduced. *Be sure to check with your physician before making any adjustments in your medication(s).*

Basic RR Techniques

Now that you have been introduced to the nature of the RR, various breathing exercises, and things you need to know before you begin RR practice, you can start learning some basic techniques that can be used to bring about the RR. It is important that you become experienced with the basic techniques before moving on to the more advanced ones.

For each of the following techniques, begin by finding yourself a quiet, comfortable position in which your body can relax.

Close your eyes (unless that is uncomfortable or unsafe—e.g., while walking in Technique 4) and begin to focus on the cue described—for example, word, breath, or creating muscle tension.

Repeatedly focus on the cue, and when you are distracted by your thoughts or pain gently guide your mind back to the focus.

RR Technique 1: Using a Focus Word or Phrase

The first RR technique is to focus on a repetitive word or short phrase on each out-breath. What word or phrase you choose is less important than its repetition. Remember that this is just a way of keeping your mind focused. You can use the number "one," or count to 10 repetitively with each breath, or count "one" on the in-breath and "two" on the out-breath.

You can also just find a sound that is comforting to say. If you have a religious or spiritual preference or practice, a short prayer or phrase can be used. I do recommend, however, that you avoid words or phrases like "Go! Go! Go!" or "I must relax!" With such phrases, your feelings of pressure to do more and more in less and less time or to perform yet another task are perpetuated. This is not the intention of RR techniques. The aim is not simply for you to do more of what you have been doing but to add a dimension of control to your life by taking the time to sit and focus, allowing your natural body wisdom to be restored.

If you find your mind wandering, gently guide it back to your focus word or phrase.

RR Technique 2: Coupling Breathing with Imagination

The second RR technique is to use your breath coupled with your imagination. This exercise is sometimes helpful to those who find focusing on their chests or abdomens too uncomfortable or anxiety-provoking.

For example, you can picture your breath coming in through your right hand and out through your left hand, or in and out through your right hand. "Breathing" through your feet can also be used. Or you can imagine the in-breath going to areas of tension such as your face, neck, or back; as you breathe out, imagine the breath and tension disappearing into the air. Each time a breath goes out, feel yourself becoming more relaxed.

RR Technique 3: Progressive Muscle Relaxation

The third RR technique is alternately to tense and relax various parts of your body. This is called "progressive muscle relaxation" and is helpful, again, for individuals who find it difficult to relax by sitting quietly.

You can reduce distraction by engaging in physical and mental focusing. For example, curl the toes of your right foot on the in-breath, and relax them on the out-breath. Next, flex your right foot back toward your head on the in-breath, and then relax the foot on the out-breath. Then straighten your right leg at the knee on the in-breath and relax the knee on the out-breath. Tense your right buttock on the in-breath and relax it on the out-breath. Repeat the sequence for the left leg, and progress up the body until all parts have been tensed and relaxed in sequence with the breath.

There are progressive relaxation tapes available that can guide you in this technique. (See "Using Relaxation Tapes" in the previous section for possible sources.)

RR Technique 4: Using Repetitive Motion

The fourth RR technique is to perform a repetitive motion while coupling your breath and mind with the motion. For instance, running, swimming, stationary bicycling, or using a treadmill can be practiced to elicit the RR, as long as your breath and mind are in sync with the movement.

As an example, let's suppose that you are walking on a treadmill. You can inhale on two steps and exhale on two steps repetitively and focus on that breath–movement rhythm. Of course, the ratio of breath to steps will depend on your level of conditioning, comfort, and speed. When you find yourself distracted from the rhythm of your breath and movement by thoughts, gently return your focus to your breath and movement.

Yoga and tai chi are also effective ways of coupling breath, mind, and motion. Such techniques involving ritualized posturing of the body were used to bring about the RR in ancient cultures.

RR Technique 5: Creating a Safe Place

Many people in pain feel betrayed by their bodies. Pain can make you feel trapped with nowhere to hide or find comfort. It is possible, by using your various senses, to recreate a safe haven in your mind; this is the fifth RR technique. Some program participants have reported strong, pleasant, and familiar odors while they are in their safe places; others have tactile (touch) sensations of warmth and softness. Everyone has different experiences. You should allow your natural sense selection to come forward—be it sound, smell, touch, sight, or a combination of the senses.

The following exercise has been one of the most beneficial versions of this fifth basic RR technique for people in pain:

1. Begin by engaging in one of the first three basic RR techniques.
2. When you are focused and relaxed, create an image in your mind that feels safe and comforting. Your safe place can be somewhere you went as a child, a pleasant vacation spot, or a place you saw in a book. It can be a favorite room in your home, your bed, or an imagined large fluffy cloud. You can move the mountains next to the seashore or create a totally bug-free forest scene . . . wherever your imagination leads. The key here is to envision a place associated with peace and comfort.
3. When you have imagined your special place, find a comfortable place to sit or lie and pass some quality time here, repeating your focus word or phrase with each breath. When you become distracted by thoughts, gently guide your awareness back to your focus.
4. Enjoy the experience!

With practice, you can recreate this image by focusing on your breath or the words "safe place" whenever you need some respite.

Advanced RR Techniques

The advanced RR techniques allow you to obtain additional results and insights. However, if you are inexperienced in achieving the RR, you may feel uncomfortable at the images that come into your head during the visualization exercise (Technique 7) if you have not first practiced and become adept at creating a safe place inside yourself. For many people in chronic pain, the pain is a beast or a big unknown, which can be quite intimidating (and scary) if not approached from a position of experience with the basic techniques. Or you may feel anxious about the instructions to create numbness and an absence of feeling in certain body areas during the self-hypnosis exercise (Technique 6). Therefore, it is recommended that you practice the advanced techniques *only* after you have had experience in eliciting the RR by means of the basic techniques, especially Technique 5 (creating a safe place).

RR Technique 6: Self-Hypnosis

The sixth RR technique is a simple self-hypnosis exercise. Begin by choosing one of the basic RR techniques that you have learned. Once you are feeling relaxed, proceed as follows:

1. Close your eyes and imagine that your right hand is becoming pleasantly warm and heavy. Each time you breathe out, the pleasant sensation of warmth and heaviness becomes greater, until your hand feels so heavy it can hardly move (unless you want it to).
2. Now feel a pleasant numbness that begins in your right thumb, then moves to your second finger, the third finger, the fourth finger, and finally the fifth finger with each out-breath. The numbness spreads to the palm of your right hand and then to the back of the hand, stopping at the wrist. It is a pleasant, warm, heavy, and numb sensation only in your right hand.
3. Either physically place your right hand on your painful area, or imagine that the numbness in your right hand is moving there. When all the numbness has been absorbed into the area of pain, return to your focus word or breath. When you are ready to end this session, transfer the numbness back to your right hand.
4. Now feel the normal sensations coming into the back of your right hand, then the palm, the fifth finger, the fourth finger, the third finger, the second finger, and the thumb. Your hand still feels warm and heavy.
5. Gradually feel your hand becoming lighter and lighter with each breath. Feel it become normal, just like your left hand.
6. Count to three and open your eyes.

The more you practice this technique, the more quickly you can develop the sensation of numbness, which can be transferred to the area of pain. You can also make your own tape with these instructions to help you master this technique.

This is a technique that can temporarily alter the pain experience. If you wish to explore hypnosis further, there are psychotherapists who have special training and certification in hypnosis who may help you identify other techniques that might suit your needs better. An inspiring story about how one person used hypnosis to control his pain can be found in *A Whole New Life* by Reynolds Price (see "Supplementary Reading" at the end of this chapter).

RR Technique 7: Visualization

RR Technique 7 is a visualization exercise in which you create and work with an image of your pain. As noted earlier, this technique should not be attempted without experience with the basic RR techniques, especially Technique 5, because many people's images of their pain can be quite frightening. If your image gets too scary, just open your eyes; remember that you have control over it.

> Gail suffered from terrible migraines that were occurring at least once a week. During the visualization exercise, she saw her pain as a red-hot ball that pulsated. When asked to modify the pain in some way, she decided to build an igloo around it, and the red ball turned blue.
>
> The next time Gail started to get her usual warning of the headache to come, she closed her eyes, imagined the red-hot ball, and then built the igloo around it until it turned blue. The headache didn't come! Gail was able to stop many of her headaches with this technique.

To begin this exercise, again, engage in one of the basic RR techniques. When you feel focused and relaxed, create an image in your mind in the following manner:

1. Imagine yourself in a meadow where the sun is shining, it's not too hot or too cool, and a gentle breeze is blowing.
2. Picture a path. As you walk along it, a sense of safety and security accompanies you. In the distance you can hear the birds singing in the trees, and you can smell the sweet scent of wildflowers. Follow the path across a bridge to a house that sits at the edge of the meadow.
3. Walk up the steps of the house and open the front door. When you walk inside, you will find a large room divided into two parts by a large wall made of clear, impenetrable plastic. This wall extends from floor to ceiling and from one end of the room to the other.
4. Make yourself comfortable and sit in front of the clear plastic wall.
5. Gather up your pain into a ball. Take this ball of pain and notice that the clear plastic wall in front of you opens up to let you drop the pain on the other side. After you have placed the pain on the other side, the wall closes up again, and the pain must remain there until you instruct it otherwise.
6. Give your pain a color, a shape, or a form. It can be a symbol of what your pain feels like, or it can be like a cartoon character.
7. Now observe its behavior. Does it bounce around, scream, or look menacing? How does being face-to-face with it make you feel?
8. Ask your pain these questions and listen to the responses:

   "Why are you here?"
   "What can I learn from you?"

"When will you go away?"
"Can we coexist together?"

9. You may ask the pain any other questions that you may have. Most people have a lot of questions to ask or things to say to their pain when given this opportunity.

10. Now think about how you might change the image of your pain in some way. For example, if it looks like a blob that is ill defined, pour it into a container and give it boundaries. You don't have to destroy it; just let your ideas and the image come freely. If it's hot, cool it down. If it's sharp, dull the edges. As you try different approaches, ask yourself how you feel about manipulating your pain. Is there any effect on your pain as you try these different approaches?

11. When you are finished asking questions and/or modifying your pain, make one of the following decisions:

Take all of the pain back.
Leave all of the pain behind the clear plastic wall.
Take part of the pain back.

12. Once you have made your decision, walk out the front door of the house and close it behind you.

13. Walk down the front steps and into the sunshine. Move along the path, over the bridge, and back into the meadow again.

14. Take the path to your safe place where you have established a haven of refuge and solace (Technique 5). Spend some time there focusing your mind and releasing any residual tension.

15. When you are finished, open your eyes.

This technique can be a very powerful emotional experience. It can be used to examine any problem, not just your pain. By removing or distancing yourself from the pain or other problem, you can get a fresh outlook, and new solutions can be explored.

Dorothy was amazed. The image before her was as gray and ominous as anything she had ever felt in all the years she had pain. It had no edges or boundaries. The pain looked like smoky wisps that crept along the edges of the clear wall, as if it were trying to find an opening to escape.

Dorothy asked it questions but received no answers. Her pain remained as elusive as it had always been. What wasn't elusive, however, was the sense of impending doom she felt whenever the pain increased.

Dorothy continued to practice this technique and always created a safe place after confronting her pain. As she began exploring the pain with her pain diary and some of the cognitive exercises (see Chapter 6), she started to see images that

(cont.)

were more concrete and defined. At first she saw a ghost, then a character that looked like the Michelin® tire man. One day she was able to pump the tire man up until it exploded into a thousand pieces.

Dorothy then felt a sense of release and relief. She realized that the fear of the pain had held her a prisoner; once she became able to face this fear, she was able to feel less controlled by it.

The use of imagery allows you to explore the nonverbal, unconscious experience of pain meanings and metaphors. It can help you make connections to other experiences or understandings that might not be reached through sequential, logical reasoning. This, in turn, can give you an entirely different perspective and attitude toward your pain and can expand your control of the pain experience.

Another way of looking at the effects of this exercise is to place your hand over your face with fingers spread apart. Your vision is impaired, and you are not able to see the back of your hand. Now, as your hand moves away from your face, you can see more details, and there is more freedom to turn your hand around to see the back and front. This distancing, like putting the pain or problem behind the plastic wall, allows you to see a greater range of options and solutions for the problems that may confront you.

Summary

Chronic Pain as Chronic Stress; The RR

- Chronic pain fits the definition of chronic stress. A chronically stressed state makes it difficult for you to reestablish homeostasis (balance) because of an exhaustion of your recuperative abilities.
- Techniques that bring about the "relaxation response" (RR) will help you restore your recuperative abilities.
- The RR is a natural bodily response, but it needs to be trained and practiced. It involves (1) focusing your mind on a repetitive phrase, word, breath, or action; and (2) adopting a passive attitude toward interfering thoughts.

Breathing; Breathing Exercises

- The key to bringing about the RR is focused awareness; breathing can be an object of that focus.
- There are two types of breathing:

  - Chest breathing—with each in-breath, your chest expands.
  - Diaphragmatic breathing—with each in-breath, your abdomen expands.

- If you are a chest breather, there are three diaphragmatic breathing exercises to help you become more aware of what parts of your body should move when you breathe diaphragmatically. If one position does not work out for you, try another.
- Once you're aware of your breathing, you can start to practice breath focusing, which encourages you to focus on the present, the here and now. By so doing, you can release tension, decrease pain, and increase control.
- Taking a moment during the day to focus on breathing can be thought of as a "mini-relaxation." Several suggestions are provided for this.

Preparing to Practice Eliciting the RR

- Minimize distractions and make yourself as comfortable as possible while you practice the RR techniques.
- Relaxation tapes can be quite helpful in learning to bring about the RR. If you plan to use relaxation tapes, don't continually change them; it is important to be consistent with your object of focus, particularly when you first begin.
- "Mind chatter" is all the thoughts going through your mind at once. This chatter, which is perfectly normal, can interrupt your meditative thoughts; however, by focusing on your repetitive word, phrase, breath, or action, you can reduce the chatter and perhaps even eliminate it temporarily.
- In the beginning, many obstacles may keep you from practicing the RR techniques; however, these techniques are critical to overcoming your pain and succeeding with this program. So, with the better interests of your health in mind, remember the following:

  - If you want to feel better, make the time to practice the techniques.
  - Your pain may get worse during practice, but you can develop your ability to focus and decrease the pain.
  - If you have difficulty with sitting still or relaxing because of physical tension, try gentle stretching or progressive muscle relaxation; if you have low self-esteem or a strong need to meet others' demands, try imagining that you are storing your worries in a basket while practicing your RR techniques.
  - If you are dealing with posttraumatic stress (e.g., sexual abuse memories), you can modify the techniques in various ways to minimize your anxiety and decrease your discomfort. Seek additional professional help if you are feeling overwhelmed.
  - If you have peculiar sensations or experiences (e.g., out-of-body experiences, dissociation) while practicing an RR technique, you may be practicing too long or too often.
  - If you have a seizure disorder, diabetes, or hypertension, specific recommendations are applicable to these disorders.

Basic RR Techniques

- Five basic RR techniques are presented.

  - Technique 1: Focus on a repetitive word or short phrase on each out-breath.
  - Technique 2: Use your breath, coupled with your imagination. Picture your in-breath going into the areas of tension, and on the out-breath, let the tension go.
  - Technique 3: Alternately tense and relax various parts of your body (this is called "progressive muscle relaxation").
  - Technique 4: Perform a repetitive motion while coupling your breath and mind with the motion.
  - Technique 5: Create a safe haven in your mind where you can leave your pain behind and go to rest.

Advanced RR Techniques

- There are two advanced RR techniques. These should be practiced only after you have become skilled in the more basic RR techniques (1–5).

  - Technique 6: This is a simple self-hypnosis technique that allows you to transfer sensations from one part of your body to another.
  - Technique 7: This is a visualization technique that allows you to place your pain behind a clear wall; give it a form; ask it questions; modify its form and study the effect on your pain; and then decide whether to take part, all, or none of it back. This technique can be a very powerful emotional experience, but it can be extremely effective; you can put any problem behind the clear plastic wall.

Exploration Tasks

1. Practice your goal-setting skills by writing out a goal that involves one of the RR techniques. Make sure that your goal meets the criteria set forth in Chapter 1—in other words, that it is a realistic behavioral task that can be measured in the steps that *you* will take to accomplish it. Here is an example:

   Goal: *Practice RR Technique 1 once a day.*

   Steps to take to reach that goal:

   A. *Take phone off hook.*

   B. *Use the recliner to maximize comfort.*

   C. *Practice as soon as I get out of bed.*

   In addition, list contingency plans. Making contingency plans is a way of troubleshooting before a problem occurs. Thinking ahead of time about what might get in the way of achieving your goal can help you develop strategies to solve the problem. Here is an example:

	Obstacles	**Solutions**
A.	_Can't relax, pain too bad_	_Listen to RR tape, practice in bathtub_
B.	_Family members disturb me_	_Hang "Do Not Disturb" sign on door_

Now it's your turn.

Goal: _____

Steps to take to reach that goal:

A. _____

B. _____

C. _____

D. _____

List contingency plans. What steps can you take to work toward insuring your success?

	Obstacles	**Solutions**
A.	_____	_____
B.	_____	_____
C.	_____	_____
D.	_____	_____

2. Practice diaphragmatic breathing as frequently as possible, both during the day and before going to sleep.

3. In the midst of tension, increased pain, or emotional distress, remember to do the following:

   A. Consciously stop and pause.
   B. Take a deep, slow breath from your diaphragm.
   C. Reflect on the situation and your choices.

4. Incorporate "mini-relaxations" into your daily routine.

   When do you do mini-relaxations? _____

   What techniques do you use? _____

   _____

   What can you do to remind yourself to do mini-relaxations throughout the day?

   _____

5. Practice an RR technique once a day for 20 minutes. In the beginning, don't be concerned with breathing diaphragmatically; just breathe your normal way. Practice the diaphragmatic breathing separately. Practice one of the basic techniques (1–5) daily for at least five weeks before moving on to the advanced techniques (6–7). Again, it is important to be comfortable with your basic technique before using the more advanced techniques.

6. Complete the RR technique diary at the back of the book. Next to each category, indicate the appropriate information about your daily practice. Use this diary for the first three weeks to reinforce practice.

Supplementary Reading

The following books provide additional information on the mind–body connection in general and the RR in particular:

Herbert Benson, *The Relaxation Response* (New York: Mass Market Paperback, 1990).
Joan Borysenko, *Minding the Body, Mending the Mind* (New York: Bantam Doubleday Dell Publications, 1993).
Patrick Fanning, *Visualization for Change* (Oakland, CA: New Harbinger Publications, 1994).
Shakti Gawain, *Creative Visualization* (New York: Bantam Books, 1983).
Thich Nhat Hanh, *The Miracle of Mindfulness: A Manual of Meditation* (Boston: Beacon Press, 1996).
Jon Kabat-Zinn, *Full Catastrophe Living: Using the Wisdom of Your Body and Mind to Face Stress, Pain, and Illness* (New York: Delacorte Press, 1990).
Reynolds Price, *A Whole New Life* (New York: Scribner, 2000).

Chapter 4

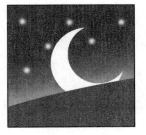

The Body–Mind Connection

Chapter 3 has explored how your mind can affect your body. Now let's take a look at how your body can affect your mind.

When you are in pain, you may tend to do the following:

- Ignore all sensation from the neck down or label all sensation as painful.
- Stop moving your body parts except when it's absolutely necessary.
- Withdraw from social interactions.
- Push yourself physically by using denial of your condition.

These attitudes and behaviors need to be challenged because they can contribute either to increased fear of activity or to excessive activity; can predispose you to decreases in muscle strength and endurance; and can sometimes even result in reinjury. They can also lead to social isolation, loneliness, and depression. One patient, John, has described all of this well in the following story.

I used to get up in the morning with the challenge of doing things as usual, in spite of my pain. Maybe today would be different. Sure, the pain was my issue, but I was also getting subtle and not-so-subtle messages from my family and friends: "It used to be so much fun when you could do this. . . . Remember when you could do

(cont.)

that? . . . When are you going back to work? It might get your mind off your problems."

I felt it was impossible to explain. No one understood. Even I had a difficult time understanding why my back continued to spasm with the least amount of activity. I was terrified of doing things for fear of making the pain worse; yet, at the same time, I was ashamed because I couldn't even keep up with the laundry. How could I ever drive a truck again—the only thing I knew how to do for a living? So each day I would push myself through the odd jobs at home and collapse at the end of the day, with the pain worse than ever.

So what did I accomplish? I became more irritable, depressed, and withdrawn. I felt trapped and alone. My children tiptoed past me as I lay on the couch, and my wife and I constantly bickered. One day I found her sobbing. She told me that she felt she had lost her best friend and husband to the pain. I made the decision there and then to seek help, and found this program.

By contrast, your body can become a resource for you, instead of something frightening that has to be ignored or pushed into submission. It can provide you with important cues and indicators on how to pace yourself and plan your activities, so that you can engage in more activities with less pain. In addition, when you learn to listen to your body, not only can you become more genuinely aware of when you are in pain—you can also actually use your body to change your mood and sensations. Finally, you can begin to engage in pleasurable activities as a means of becoming more involved with life again. This chapter will show you how to do all these things.

Increasing Activities

Pain can prevent you from moving comfortably. It can make work and pleasurable activities more difficult, if not downright impossible. Through keeping your diary, you may be starting to see how your pain is influenced by your activities and your activities altered by your pain. Keeping active while in pain requires consideration of three factors:

- Pacing
- Adaptation
- Delegation

Pacing is about conserving your energy over the long haul and not letting the stress of pain and overactivity decrease it. Instead of "sprinting" through an activity, you "walk." Instead of working harder, you work smarter. This approach can serve two purposes. One, you are more likely to get a task done, and two, you can get it done without necessarily increasing your pain and suffering. The processes that trigger increases in pain, such as fatigue and spasm, may be reduced by pacing activities, because the body isn't pushed to exhaustion. Pushing yourself to the point of exhaustion can increase tension, inflammation, and nerve irritation. Pacing has to do with observing that certain positions (such as sitting or standing) or certain activities (such as vacuuming or combing your hair) may increase your pain. For example, becoming aware of how long you can stand before your pain goes from a "4" to a "6" (on the 0–10 scale, ranging from 0 = no pain to 10 = severe pain) can give you an idea of how long you can stand to do the dishes before you sit and pay your bills. You then note how long you are sitting before the pain goes back down to "4." Once you have the idea, you can alternate sitting with standing activities, get more accomplished, and not increase your pain and exhaustion. It's recommended that you use a timer or other cueing device so that the temptation to pay one more bill or do one more dish is limited. Let's take a look at John's usual day before starting this program and his usual day now, as an example.

Then		Now	
9 A.M.	Get up	7 A.M.	Get up
	Pain sensation = 6 **Emotional response = 7**		**Pain sensation = 5** **Emotional response = 3**
9:30 A.M.	Breakfast	7:30 A.M.	Stretching, relaxation technique
10:30 A.M.	Do the dishes, watch TV	8:30 A.M.	Shower, get dressed
11 A.M.	Lie down	9 A.M.	Get bills together to pay
1 P.M.	Get up and eat lunch	9:15 A.M.	Wash dishes for 10 minutes
1:30 P.M.	Work on the car (Pain = 7)	9:25 A.M.	Pay bills for 15 minutes
3:00 P.M.	Pick up children	9:40 A.M.	Bring laundry down in four small bundles
4:30 P.M.	Eat dinner		
5:00 P.M.	Watch TV	10 A.M.	Log on Internet for support group
7:00 P.M.	Go to bed		
	Pain sensation = 8 **Emotional response = 7**	10:20 A.M.	Start wash in washing machine
		11 A.M.	Finish bills
		11:30 A.M.	Finish dishes
		Noon	Eat lunch
		12:30 P.M.	Put wet clothes in dryer
		1:00 P.M.	Peel vegetables for dinner
		1:45 P.M.	Take dry clothes out of dryer
		2:15 P.M.	Fold clothes while sitting
		3 P.M.	Pick up children at school
		3:15–6 P.M.	Watch soccer game
		6:15 P.M.	Set table

(cont.)

Then	Now	
	6:30 P.M.	Eat dinner
	7:00 P.M.	Stretches
	7:30 P.M.	Help children with homework
	9:00 P.M.	Read bedtime story
	9:30 P.M.	Hot shower and bed
		Pain sensation = 5
		Emotional response = 3

Adaptation is about finding new ways to accomplish old tasks or using devices to help do routine activities. For example, there is no rule that dishes need to be done in the sink or the clothes folded while standing if standing is too painful. Sitting while using a dishpan at the kitchen table or folding clothes is quite all right! Putting a bench in the shower stall or bathtub can let you sit and scrub, using shoes with Velcro clasps and putting large handle grips on stirring spoons and pens are all devices to make your life more comfortable. Such devices and ideas can be obtained from your local hospital's occupational therapy department and by sharing ideas with participants in local pain support groups or on the Internet.

Delegation is another way of conserving your energy. It's like job sharing. "If you carry the laundry upstairs, I'll fold it." "If you get the bills together, I'll pay them."

"You clean the bathrooms, I'll pick up the living room." Entertain by hosting potlucks—everyone brings a dish. Tell them that if they volunteer to wash or dry dishes, they don't have to prepare anything! Can't do a certain task? Ask a friend. They may have something you can do for them in return—and don't forget to pace!

Pacing, adaptation, and delegation allow you the most flexibility while acknowledging that your pain is real but can be incorporated into your life.

Dealing with Difficulties in Changing the Way You Do Your Activities

You may, of course, be able to think of any number of reasons for not pacing yourself or altering your routines:

"I don't do enough as it is. How can I take a break?"

"I have to do things like everyone else, or at least like my mother [or father] did."

"I'm too busy to take a break. What will my family do?"

"I can't ask for help, understanding, or a change in schedule."

"My pain is always the same no matter what I do."

It may be difficult for you to take the lead in deciding what you can and cannot do (instead of living up to others' expectations). As this book states repeatedly, however, it is absolutely essential that *you* take control. No one else can judge what you are able or not able to do.

The following story shows why it's so important to examine what you do and why you do it.

A woman was busy fixing a Sunday pot roast. She cut off the ends of the roast in her preparation. Her daughter watched as she did this and asked why she cut the ends off the roast.

"Well," she said after some contemplation, "that's how my mother used to prepare it. Let's call Grammy and ask her."

She called her mother and asked, "Why do you cut the ends off a pot roast?"

Her mother replied, "Hmmm. . . . I guess I never thought about it before because my mother, your grandmother, always did it."

Curious now as to what the answer might be, the woman called her grandmother to solve this culinary mystery. In response to the inquiry from her granddaughter, the grandmother laughed and laughed. "I used to cut off the ends of the pot roast because it was always too big to fit into the tiny roasting pan that fit in my little oven of 50 years ago!"

By examining what you do, you can decide what you want to keep and what you want to discard—like the ends of a pot roast. I recommend that once you have determined what *you need* (as opposed to what others expect) by way of pacing your activities as outlined above, you should notify those around you. Other people will generally be supportive of alterations in your routines if they are advised of the reasons and the intent. They certainly will respond to your being in a better mood and in less discomfort.

Martha decided that she could stand to do dishes at the sink for only five minutes before she needed to sit down. She arranged to use her oven timer to cue her when the five minutes were up. She also arranged to have some stationery and her address book on the kitchen table, so that she could catch up on correspondence; she would do this for 10 minutes while she sat and "rested." At first the other members of her family did not understand. Some wondered why she was "goofing off" in this way; others kept trying to finish the dishes for her when they saw her sit down. Martha was able to tell them that this was what she needed to do for herself, and reminded them (and herself) that there was no rule limiting dishwashing to any specific period of time. She felt better about accomplishing this task by herself, and because of her pacing she experienced no increase in pain. With this success, she was able to determine the time and positioning requirements for the other tasks she wanted to accomplish.

Working Outside the Home

If you are still working outside the home or contemplating return to work, it is important to stick to a routine that includes taking care of yourself. Regular sleep hours, exercise, good nutrition, and stress management are important for general health, as well as for maintaining a work capacity, when you have chronic pain. Returning to work can mean confronting the fears of reinjury or increased pain or the unknowns of working while in pain. Strategies covered in future chapters will address these challenges. In addition, this may be the opportunity to consider self-employment ideas so that the maximum flexibility can be assured for your workday pacing.

Many people complain that pacing themselves at home is all well and good, but at work, "it's impossible!" Actually, the same ideas can be applied in the workplace environment, but doing so may take a little more brainstorming or creative problem solving. For one thing, there are external time pressures at work; for another, pacing yourself in the workplace may involve synchronizing your efforts with the work of other people. I generally recommend that once you identify the various work tasks and their time and positioning requirements, you should create a flow chart or diagram of how you can perform these tasks throughout the day using the pacing routine. This should include alternating between sitting and standing tasks, as well as between tasks you can do individually and those that involve other people.

Using a Post-it® Note to describe each task and its time and positioning requirements, and then moving the notes around on a large piece of paper, may help you with organizing your day.

Other strategies can include setting the timer on the computer and doing a minute of stretching every hour, or bringing a cot to lie on while listening at board or staff meetings. Or you may need to work with an occupational therapist to determine job modifications or the need for adaptive equipment. Again, letting those around you know that you have specific needs and that certain approaches work best for you allows you to assert choice. It also gives the clear message that you do not require being rescued and that the situation is under control. For the many people around you who are at a loss as to what to do and would like to help, the guidelines you give them can enable them to help you and work with you more effectively.

Common Problems When Becoming Active

If you find yourself needing hours or a whole day to recover in between activities, you have probably not stopped an activity soon enough and just need to practice responding earlier to increases in tightness, fatigue, and pain. Your pain diary will help you fine-tune your pain sensation awareness, as will some exercises described later in this chapter.

If you find yourself experiencing delays in pain increases—for example, you clean out the garage one day without excessive pain, but the next day you ache all over even more—then you are probably experiencing the effects of "deconditioning." Deconditioning is a combination of decreased muscle strength and endurance that occurs as a result of not having a regular exercise routine. This is a common problem for patients with chronic pain. A regular exercise/conditioning program may be of great value in such circumstances, as it will allow you to increase your endurance and limit muscle fatigue. Such a program may involve walking, swimming, using a stationary bicycle or treadmill, or practicing tai chi or yoga (see "Aerobic Exercise," below). The choice, of course, depends on where you are having pain and what your physical limitations are.

Remember, too, that your level of pain may not *necessarily* correlate with your ability to function. Many people are able to increase their activity and functional level without necessarily increasing their pain. Once you go through the soreness and tightness that are normal and expectable consequences of starting an exercise or activity routine, you may find yourself more active but in no more pain than you were before. Again, the sensation-labeling exercises described later in the chapter may help you to discriminate between these normal feelings and pain that serves as a danger signal. The value in considering all of this is that you may be able to become more active in spite of the pain and without fear of doing harm, which inhibits many of the activities of people experiencing chronic pain.

Time Management

In order to pace, adapt, and delegate effectively, it's important to take a look at all that you do during the course of a day. That way you can see exactly how much time you spend on certain activities. Putting a routine schedule into your life can make you feel useful again. Getting up and going to bed at the same time also helps establish a natural body rhythm. Having your day planned can help you accomplish your tasks and insures that pacing is not an afterthought. You may also find it very helpful to prepare a backup plan in advance for managing those inevitable flare-up days (see Chapter 10). Even if you can't work outside the home, consider volunteering. You can apply the pacing activities here to help you be successful and reap the good feelings associated with helping others.

The Time Pie

An exercise that is helpful in determining what you do during a day is to draw a pie chart (or "time pie"). Break up your 24-hour day into the time periods your different activities require. That is, identify each activity as a wedge in the time pie. For example, you may have wedges for sleeping, working on the job, meeting with friends, talking on the phone, reading, watching TV, doing housework, playing with the kids, and so on. This is a nice way to graphically display what really takes place each day—something most people rarely think about. If each day of your week is different, then make seven time pies; if your weekdays are different from your weekends, make two time pies—one for weekdays and one for weekends. Draw your pie(s) in the space provided on the following page.

Now draw a pie that you would find more acceptable, given your pain level and what you are learning. Ask yourself the following questions, and write down your answers:

1. How many hours of my day are devoted to meeting others' needs? _____

2. Do all of these activities really need my involvement? _____

3. What activities can I share with or assign to the person or persons who are currently requiring my time? _____

4. What activities that I am not currently pursuing would I like to add to (or put back into) my routine? _____

5. What steps can I take to make my present pie into a more acceptable pie? _____

_____

_____

Use this space to draw your time pies—both your current one(s) and your ideal one:

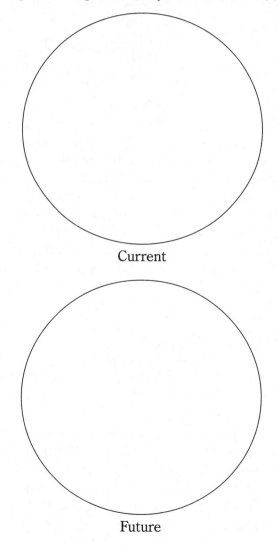

Current

Future

True Confessions: Choosing Your Activities Consciously

Most people derive their sense of personal worth from the things they do. Therefore, it is important to realize how you define yourself through your activities, because this will affect your choices in regard to activity planning and time management. For example, you may find it very difficult not to do all the tasks for your family. I'll never forget one patient who complained about how she had to get up early every morning to pack lunches for her children. When I inquired about their ages, thinking that if they were teenagers they might be old enough to pack their own lunches, she replied, "Oh, they're 26 and 28 years old!" Although altruism is ennobling, it's not healthy for you or for others if you do your helping mindlessly or with secret bitterness. Helping mindlessly can contribute to hurting yourself through overdoing, and doing for others because you feel you "have to" rather than because you "want to" can create resentment and feelings of being used and abused.

Another point you may wish to consider is that pain can be used as an excuse not to do things people don't want to do, as well as something that prevents them from doing the things they do want to do. Pain can also be used to control others and elicit attention that people might not otherwise get. Sometimes people in chronic pain feel guilty when they become aware of such behaviors in themselves. I find that such behaviors are usually unconscious and are the result of pain's effectiveness as a means of both obtaining attention and avoiding undesirable obligations. Understanding how you incorporate your pain experience into your life can help you choose which behaviors you may want to explore further or avoid.

You really do have choices. This is your opportunity to explore a new you. It's okay to say "no." It's okay to say "yes." For now, it's enough that you make all of your choices conscious. If you choose to continue a certain activity or behavior, do it with your commitment and *your* choice: Own it.

Listening to Your Body

As noted at the beginning of this chapter, your body can be the source of important cues. By becoming aware of your body's messages, you can avoid potential problems and even soothe yourself. This section presents a series of exercises in learning to listen to your body. Read through the exercises once, then try them.

The following exercises will help you do or learn the following:

- Gently stretch your muscles.
- Gently move your limbs through their range of motion.
- Isolate muscle tension.
- Relabel sensations.
- Use breathing to release tension.
- Develop body awareness.
- Allow yourself to experience the pleasant, energizing feelings associated with simple exercise.

If your muscles are not stretched and your limbs do not go through their range of motion, then your stiffness, tightness, and tension will increase, especially upon rising in the morning. If you limit your "exercise" to the movement involved in your daily chores, you will be likely to overextend tight muscles. Doing slow, purposeful exercises, such as the ones explained here, will help minimize injury.

If any of the following movements increases your pain, you can modify the movement so that a gentle stretch is obtained with no increase in pain. If you are unable to stretch a limb gently, then skip it (or imagine yourself doing the stretch in your mind) and go on to the next limb.

Labeling Sensations in Your Legs

1. Sit comfortably in a chair.
2. Point your right foot in front of you and lift it off the ground. Keep breathing slowly and regularly. How would you describe the sensation you feel? Tightness, stretching, burning, aching? (Avoid using the word "pain" or "it hurts"; these terms are too vague. Learning to describe the sensation more accurately may give you clues as to its cause and effect, which may lead to more specific remedies.) Also, where exactly do you feel these sensations? Front of lower leg, across the top of the foot, around the knee?
3. Now, as you point your right foot, become aware of the tension you may have placed in your left leg, arms, or face as you create the stretch. Make sure that only the right leg is tense, and relax the other parts of your body. Keep breathing slowly and regularly.
4. Take a deep breath. On the out-breath, release the tension in your right leg, letting the foot rest once again on the floor.
5. Close your eyes. How does your right leg feel compared with the left leg? Warm, tingling, tired, vibrant?
6. Now point your left foot in front of you and lift it off the ground. Make sure you don't get your arms or face involved in creating the tension, and keep breathing regularly. What sensations do you feel? Tightness, stretching, burning, aching?
7. Take a deep breath. On the out -breath, release the tension in your left leg, letting the foot rest once again on the floor.
8. Close your eyes and compare how your right and left legs feel now.

Labeling Sensations in Your Arms

While exercising your arms, make sure that your legs and face are not involved in the tension. And, once again, be sure to keep breathing slowly and regularly.

1. Make a fist with your right hand and hold your right arm out in front of you. How would you describe the sensations you feel? Where do you feel them?
2. Take a deep breath. On the out-breath, relax your fist and let the tension go. How does your right arm feel compared with the left one?

3. Now make a fist with your left hand and hold your left arm out in front of you. What sensations do you feel? Where do you feel them?
4. Take a deep breath. On the out-breath, relax your fist and let the tension go. How does your left arm feel compared with the right one?

Labeling Sensations in Your Shoulders

Like the other exercises, this exercise should be done slowly, accompanied by nice deep breaths.

1. Put the fingertips from both hands on their respective shoulders.
2. Raise your elbows out from your sides, and rotate the elbows as if you are drawing circles in the air.
3. Move your elbows in circles with each breath, so that each complete circle takes one slow breath. Make sure that the tension is only in your shoulders and upper back.
4. Draw circles in one direction five times, then draw circles in the other direction five times.
5. Take a deep breath. On the out-breath, let your hands fall gently back into your lap.
6. Close your eyes and see whether you can distinguish any sensation (tired, achy, vibrant, burning?) in your upper back, shoulders, and neck.

Labeling Sensations in Your Face

As in the previous exercises, breathing is very important; however, it may be a bit more difficult in this case because of the facial movements involved.

1. Imagine that you have just bitten into a lemon, and wrinkle your face.
2. Feel the tension in your face, and check to see whether the rest of your body is relaxed.
3. Keep breathing slowly and regularly. (This may be hard to do through a wrinkled nose!)
4. Take a deep breath. On the out-breath, relax your face.
5. Close your eyes. Now check out your whole body by doing a "body sweep." That is, use your mind like a flashlight and shine it on each part of your body that you have just stretched. Release any residual tension by breathing into the tense area and breathing out the tension. How do you feel?

Rating Your Pain

The following exercise will help you to translate physical sensation into numbers. You may find this especially helpful if you have had any difficulty in giving your pain a numerical rating in your pain diary.

Use a scale of 0 to 10 when making a fist, with 0 being the loosest fist and 10 being the tightest fist. When you get to the end of these instructions, do the exercise before you continue.

1. Make a number 5 fist. How would you describe the sensations you feel? Where do you feel them?
2. Relax the fist.
3. Now make a number 2 fist. What sensations do you feel? Where do you feel them? What makes the number 2 fist different from the number 5 fist?
4. Relax the fist.
5. Now make a number 9 fist. What sensations do you feel? Where do you feel them? What makes the number 9 fist different from the number 5 fist?
6. Relax the fist.

Be sure to try this exercise before you read on.

The following are some comments made by patients who did this exercise:

"Sensation is relative, and so is pain."

"A number 2 pain is more tolerable than a number 5 pain, but even a number 5 pain is tolerable compared to a number 9 pain."

"A number 2 pain is more localized, with the pain spreading away from the original painful area as the rating goes higher. . . . The higher the number given the pain, the more dysfunction is associated with it, both physically and emotionally."

A lot of the spreading of pain has to do with the additional tension or breath holding that takes place in response to pain—as in the first breath-focusing exercise in Chapter 3 (the fist–breath exercise). The pain sensation becomes the focal point of attention, which in turn increases the awareness, which increases the distress, which increases the tension, and so on and on. Instead, you can take a deep breath and breathe out slowly.

Apply this to your own pain rating. See whether you can discern the subtleties of what you once thought to be only one sensation but may in fact be many. Once you develop an awareness of the tension that may be resulting from holding your breath or breathing shallowly, as well as of the normal sensations of tightness and "good hurts" that are part of beginning an exercise routine, you will be in a much better position to do activities and exercises safely. (Continued practice with an RR technique will also help fine-tune this skill.) If all you can do on a regular basis are these simple sensation-labeling exercises, they will help keep your muscles, bones, and joints healthy.

Using Your Body to Change Your Mood

Patients sometimes confide in me that they no longer tell their friends or family members when they are having a bad day. These are the same people sitting in front of me with their shoulders sagging and brows tense. They grimace as they frequently change positions, and they sigh a lot. Who's kidding whom?

People communicate in many ways that have nothing to do with their words, and you are no exception. These subtle behaviors are definite communications with the outside world, and sometimes the outside world is listening. But sometimes being subtle and less than direct allows those around you to ignore what they feel powerless to change, or to interpret your actions or behaviors incorrectly. People judge by appearances, and most people cannot imagine living with chronic pain. Giving mixed messages with your body and your words causes more confusion for you and for those watching you. When you assume certain body postures and facial expressions such as the ones just described, you may be reinforcing negative emotions and making your situation even worse than it already is.

Try this simple exercise:

1. Raise your eyebrows and show your teeth.
2. Hold this posture for 30 seconds. What kinds of thoughts pass through your mind? (Ignore the ones that say you must look goofy.)
3. Relax.
4. Now bring your eyebrows together and clench your jaw and fists. What are you thinking now?

The first expression is usually associated with happiness, and the second one with anger and rage. How did you feel? Psychologist Paul Ekman and his colleagues (see "Supplementary Reading") have demonstrated that assuming these facial expressions is associated with the mood-specific physiological changes of sadness, happiness, and anger. When you get more of your body involved in creating these expressions, the emotional connection is even greater.

Now for the final exercise in this chapter. This may be a bit uncomfortable for you, but it is important and helps you get in touch with your body–mind connection. If the first position is too difficult, try it in bed rather than in a chair, and assume a "fetal" position—knees to chest, head down toward chest.

1. Sit in a chair.
2. Bend your head down, hunch your shoulders, cross your arms in front of you, and cross your legs.
3. Close your eyes for one minute. What do you *feel* emotionally? Do not use the word "pain," and stick to descriptions of emotions, not descriptions of physical sensations.
4. Relax.
5. Now stand up and place your feet apart, approximately the width of your hips.
6. Keep your shoulders back, your head high, your face to the front, and your arms down with the palms facing forward.
7. Close your eyes. What do you *feel* now?

The first position is associated with a wide range of feelings, such as the following:

- Sadness
- Fear
- Defenselessness
- Need for safety
- Need for security

The second position is usually associated with these feelings:

- Empowerment
- Being exposed
- Sense of control
- Positive attitude

Clearly, just like your pain perceptions, the wide range of responses to body posture reflects complex body–mind language that you have automatically learned over the years. This is why people will sometimes experience strong emotional reactions during massage therapy or certain physical therapy procedures. This muscular imprinting of emotions and old habits is also the principle behind various movement therapies, Feldenkrais and Alexander techniques in particular.

When you are feeling sad, try to change your facial expression and body posture to ones associated with joy and happiness. See how difficult it is to continue feeling sad. Or, if you're committed to suffering for the moment, exaggerate your suffering expression and posture even more. Don't forget to add a few moans. If you do this consciously, you may be surprised at the results. Misery loves company, even if it's your own.

Aerobic Exercise

Aerobic exercise at least three times a week can help improve your general health, particularly your heart and lung function. It can also help with weight control. Aerobic exercise ("aerobic" means literally "requires oxygen") elevates heart rate through sustained movements of the body at moderate intensity. Activities such as brisk walking, swimming, and stationary bicycling are considered aerobic exercise. There is a long list of diseases associated with a sedentary lifestyle—for example, heart disease, obesity, and osteoporosis. The risk of developing these disorders can be reduced by regular aerobic exercise. Just because you're in pain doesn't mean you need to neglect your overall health and well-being. (Quite the contrary, in fact.)

Physiatrist James Rainville and others have found that pain perception and the ability to engage in certain activities are not always matched (particularly in patients with low back pain), probably because most perceptions are subjective. A lot of people who have pain are afraid to move because they fear that the pain will increase and that they will harm themselves further. However, by not moving, stretching, or engaging in some type of exercise, they are placing themselves at greater risk for reinjury or becoming even more out of shape. Regular exercise may also be effective in reducing your pain, as demonstrated in arthritis patients (see Minor and Sanford in "Supplementary Reading"). If you exercise carefully and slowly, you are not likely to make your condition worse. Consult your physician or a physical therapist if you have specific questions regarding what you can do and how you should proceed. Those of you with low back pain may find the physical activity and exercise descriptions in *The Back Pain Helpbook* beneficial (see "Supplementary Reading").

For people in pain, water exercises can be especially relaxing, because about 70% of the effects of gravity are lost in water. Movement in water offers the opportunity to strengthen muscles, stretch, and increase heart and lung function. The Arthritis Foundation sponsors water aerobic programs all across the United States. Contact the Arthritis Foundation in your state for details. Since movement is so much easier in water, however, you may be tempted to exercise longer and harder. It's always best to start out doing much less than you think you can do and gradually increasing the length or intensity of your water exercise as you progress.

Other forms of exercise that can give you a good aerobic workout include the following:

- Riding a stationary bike.
- Walking on a treadmill.
- Using indoor cross-country ski equipment.
- Walking. (This is a particularly good exercise, as it's inexpensive and can be done almost anywhere, indoors or outdoors.)
- Yoga or tai chi. (These exercises are helpful to patients in pain, because they are slow, purposeful, and coordinated with breathing. They can also be easily adapted for those with limited movement. It is important, however, to get individual instruction and work with an instructor who can modify the positions to meet your needs.)

My colleagues and I strongly encourage individuals in chronic pain to do some type of aerobic, stretching, and strengthening exercise on a regular basis, if at all possible, for the health of their bodies and minds.

Pleasurable Activities

Little Things

Most of us miss out
on life's big prizes.
The Pulitzer. The Nobel. Oscars. Tonys. Emmys.
But we're all eligible for
life's small pleasures.
A pat on the back.

A kiss
behind the ear.
A four-pound bass.
A full moon.
An empty parking space.
A crackling fire. A great meal. A glorious sunset.
Hot soup.
Cold beer.
Don't fret about copping life's grand awards.
Enjoy its tiny delights.
There are plenty for all of us.

—Anonymous

Pleasurable activities should constitute a normal part of life, but for many living with chronic pain, they simply don't. Some patients feel so bad about their pain and their lack of a "productive life" that they cannot engage in, or even admit wanting to engage in, pleasurable activities. They don't feel that they deserve any pleasure.

The truth of the matter, however, is that if you can't engage in some pleasurable activity, any suggestions to increase your general activities will be more difficult. It's easier to start becoming involved in life again by doing something pleasurable. (See the book *Healthy Pleasures* in the "Supplementary Reading" section at the end of this chapter.)

There are any number of ways to pursue pleasurable activities, but let's just say that you should do something purposeful, conscious, and enjoyable on a regular basis. It can be something as simple as feeding the birds, watching the sunset, or observing children at play. It doesn't have to be an outing, though it can be. It's often the little things in life that make our days meaningful. The key here is to make it *conscious and purposeful.* As the philosopher Epictetus (circa A.D. 55–135) said, "Practice yourself, for heaven's sake, in little things; and thence proceed to greater." In addition, take an active part in creating your own happiness. Participating in someone else's idea of a pleasurable activity doesn't count unless you are taking pleasure from that person's pleasure or enjoying the activity yourself. Also, when you have completed your pleasurable activity, do not spend 10 minutes describing how miserable you were and apologizing for engaging in it. There is something to be said for counting your blessings.

It's possible that you may be intimidated by having to seek out a pleasurable activity. Sometimes substituting the word "satisfaction" or "beauty" instead of pleasure helps. Look for something that you can feel satisfied with or that has a beauty you can identify.

Once you have discovered and enjoyed a pleasurable activity, try sharing it with someone. For example, if you just saw a beautiful sunrise on your way to work, you could share it with a colleague. People, it seems, are always willing to give a litany of their disappointments and bad news, but it is amazing how contagious and uplifting the sharing of pleasures can be. It's also a lovely way to begin dinner conversation. Let everyone have a turn to report a little pleasure they noted that day. Life has a whole different feel to it when you become an active participant.

In short, it's okay to do something nice and pleasurable for yourself. You're worth it!

Summary

Increasing Activities

- Keeping active while in pain requires consideration of pacing, adaptation, and delegation.
- When the body is not in a constant state of exhaustion, it has a chance to recuperate more effectively.

Time Management

- Drawing a "time pie" helps you identify your daily activities and the time spent on them; it provides you with a graphic depiction of how you spend each day.
- Take a look at each activity, and examine why you engage in it.
- Consider asking for assistance from others who are capable of helping.

Listening to Your Body

- Your body can be the source of important cues; by listening to your body and labeling your sensations, you can develop an awareness of your body that will allow you to increase your activity level safely and to intervene in the development of tension earlier than you otherwise would.
- Gentle stretching exercises, involving moving your limbs through their range of motion, will help you to label sensations in various parts of your body.
- The exercises also help relieve the stress, tension, and stiffness usually associated with inactivity.
- Learning not to label all body sensations as painful will help you to pace activities, such as exercise, more realistically.

Using Your Body to Change Your Mood

- Body postures and facial expressions can either reinforce negative emotions or uplift your spirits.
- By paying attention to how your body is communicating with the outside world as well as with your internal world, you have the power to change how you feel.

Aerobic Exercise

- Aerobic exercise at least three times a week can help improve your general health, particularly your heart and lungs; it can also help with weight control.
- Water exercises are particularly helpful, because about 70% of the effects of gravity are lost in water.

- Other types of exercise that can give you a good workout include the following:
  - Riding a stationary bike
  - Walking on a treadmill
  - Using indoor cross-country ski equipment
  - Walking
  - Yoga or tai chi

Pleasurable Activities

- Pleasurable activities should be conscious and purposeful. They help you become involved in your surroundings and make your days meaningful.
- Once you have discovered a pleasurable activity, share it with someone.
- You deserve to engage in pleasurable activities for your psychological and physical health.

Exploration Tasks

1. Reread this chapter and do the various exercises as they are presented, if you have not already done so.

2. Write out a goal that you want to accomplish related to this chapter. As in earlier goal-setting exercises, make sure your goal is a behavioral task that you can measure in terms of the steps that *you* will take to accomplish it. Here is an example:

Goal: *Do the stretches described in the section "Listening to Your Body" once a day.*

Steps to take to reach that goal:

A. *Use the kitchen chair.*

B. *Place the instructions on a second chair beside me.*

C. *Do the stretches just before I do my RR technique.*

Now it's your turn.

Goal: _____

Steps to take to reach that goal:

A. _____

B. _____

C. _____

D. _____

Now list contingency plans. That is, identify what obstacles might get in the way of your accomplishing this goal. What solutions can you devise to work toward insuring the success of this goal? See Chapter 3 ("The Mind–Body Connection") for an explanation of contingency plans if you've forgotten.

	Obstacles	**Solutions**
A.	_____	_____
B.	_____	_____
C.	_____	_____
D.	_____	_____

3. Identify some type of stretching exercise that you can do daily. What will you do?

   How often will you be able to do it? _____

4. Identify some type of aerobic exercise that you can do at least three times a week.

   What will you do? _____

   How often will you be able to do it? _____

5. Identify some type of strengthening program that you can do three times per week. This can involve isometrics with an elasticized cord for that purpose, free weights, or weight machines. A good resource for women (and men) is *Strong Women Stay Young* (see "Supplementary Reading"). Ask your medical professional for recommendations or a physical therapy referral for a safe exercise program for you to do that takes your physical limitations (not necessarily your pain) into consideration.

   What will you do? _____

   How often will you be able to do it? _____

6. Continue with one of the basic RR techniques (see Chapter 3) at least once a day.

7. Choose a pleasurable activity and engage in it once a week at a minimum. Share it with someone.

   List some pleasurable activities that you might like to try:

   _____

   _____

   _____

   _____

   (Don't forget the spontaneous pleasures, like listening to children's laughter or reveling in a sunny day.)

8. If your pain increases with activities or certain postures during your daily activities, take some time to fill out the "Increasing Activities Worksheet" at the end of this book. Determine your average daily level of pain from your daily diary sheet as your baseline pain.

   Now make a list of activities that increase and decrease your pain. What are the common threads identifying each category? Posture? Length of time? Fatigue? Motivation? What happens if you alternate the activities that increase pain with those that decrease pain? Can you fine-tune any of the activities to make them easier to do in bits, like John did (e.g., dividing the laundry to carry downstairs into four smaller bundles)?

Remember, the goal is to keep active while not significantly increasing the pain. This takes doing your daily routine differently, but a lot can still be accomplished nonetheless.

Beware of telling yourself, "Just one more dish [minute, task, etc.] before stopping." Use external cues such as timers to dictate when the time is up and/or your position needs to be changed.

As you continue working with the entire program, you will need to reassess your routine periodically, because your endurance may increase as your tension decreases. Make copies of the pacing activities worksheet at the back of the book so that you can reassess your times monthly.

Supplementary Reading

The following books and articles provide additional information on exercise, body awareness, and healthy pleasures:

Lorna Bell and Eudora Seyfer, *Gentle Yoga* (Berkeley, CA: Celestial Arts, 1987).

Paul Ekman, Robert Levenson, and Wallace Friesen, "Autonomic Nervous System Activity Distinguishes among Emotions," *Science, 221*: 1208–1210, 1983.

Carol Krucoff, Mitchell Krucoff, and Adam Brill, *Healing Moves: How to Cure, Relieve, and Prevent Common Ailments with Exercise* (New York: Crown Publishers, 2000).

Kate Lorig, James Fries, and Maureen Gecht, *The Arthritis Helpbook: A Tested Self-Management Program for Coping with Arthritis and Fibromyalgia* (Reading, MA: Perseus Books, 2000).

M. A. Minor and M. K. Sanford, "Physical Interventions in the Management of Pain in Arthritis," *Arthritis Care and Research 6*: 197–206, 1993.

James Moore, Kate Lorig, Michael VanKorff, Virginia Gonzalez, and Diane Laurent, *The Back Pain Helpbook* (Reading, MA: Perseus Books, 1999).

Miriam Nelson, Wendy Wray, and Sarah Wernick, *Strong Women Stay Young* (New York: Bantam Doubleday Dell Publications, 2000).

Robert Ornstein and David Sobel, *Healthy Pleasures* (Reading, MA: Perseus Books, 1990).

James Rainville, David Ahern, Linda Phalen, Lisa Childs, and Robin Sutherland, "The Association of Pain with Physical Activities in Chronic Low Back Pain," *Spine, 17*: 1060–1064, 1992.

Chapter 5

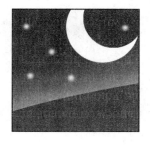

The Power of the Mind

My anxiety stems from a feeling that no one is there to take care of me. If I give in to the pain, react the way I really feel, my world will fall apart, I won't have any income, my husband will leave, no one will like me. I am worried all the time about getting things done, screwing things up, letting others down, making other people angry. I need to escape. I need to be released from these worries by having someone say: "Start over. Build a life based on what you want, and let the other chips fall where they may." If I did that, what if I couldn't figure out what I wanted? What if I was still unhappy and without a husband, job, or money?

—*Passage from a writing exercise on pain by Joan, a patient*

Harnessing the Power of the Mind: Cognitive Techniques

We know that certain ways of thinking—for example, catastrophizing, denial, avoidance, and wishful thinking—are commonly associated with disability in chronic pain and with poor coping in stressful times. Many of these ways of thinking have to do with feeling out of control. We also know that these thinking patterns can be changed to ones that enhance self-control, and that is why we strongly encourage you to take the following pages to heart.

People who catastrophize see whatever happens to them as self-defeating ("It's awful and I can't take it anymore"). Denial ("Nothing wrong with me") and avoidance ("If I don't move at all, I'll be all right") allow people to ignore their need to pace activities or increase their dysfunction. In wishful thinking, an individual may postpone acting on the need for pain management by saying to him- or herself, "Maybe my pain will be gone soon."

We know from research that certain beliefs about pain—for example, "It's mysterious and unknowable," "What happens to me is determined by chance," or "Whatever happens to me is out of my control and will defeat me"—are all associated with increased negative emotions and disability. A healthy approach to chronic pain treatment needs to include information about pain and exploration of the relationships of thoughts, feelings, and beliefs to make it all less mysterious. This exploration can serve to take advantage of the complex mind–body experience of pain. It can also help repair damaged self-esteem, create new directions, and help you gain control over your pain.

The mind, the source of thoughts and feelings, gives meaning to our experiences, including pain. A self-defeated, hopeless frame of mind will most likely contribute to the interpretation of pain signals in a negative way, increasing distress and despair. The mind can be seen as a filter through which the pain signal passes and is either dampened or magnified in intensity. Your pain experience may not be as grim or intense on a sunny, warm day or when someone has said "I love you" or when you have received a letter from a friend you've been missing as it is on a rainy, cold day when no one has called or written you in weeks and you have nothing to do.

You have already begun to harness the power of the mind with your practice of the RR techniques (see Chapter 3). The work described in this chapter will ask you to explore some of the things that determine how you see the world around you and interpret what happens to you. The techniques presented here are called "cognitive" techniques ("cognitive" is derived from "cognition," which means "knowing" or "thinking"). A good place to begin is by examining the content of your thoughts and their relation to how you feel emotionally.

Self-Talk or Automatic Thoughts

One of the most helpful tools for changing the way you think is to listen to what you say to yourself as you respond to events, physically, emotionally, and socially. We call this "self-talk." This approach is based on the premise that many moods, emotions, and feelings are sustained, if not created, by self-talk. If you change the way you talk to yourself, you can actually change how you feel.

For example, reread the passage from Joan's writing exercise presented at the beginning of this chapter. What do your feel? Do you sense the panic, anxiety, and fear that tormented this woman, just by reading her written thoughts? If you do, it may give you some indication of the power of thoughts. If you find yourself judging the content instead, you may benefit from reading the section on empathy in the next chapter.

Self-talk can accompany both negative and positive emotions. Some people are thought to engage routinely in positive self-talk (the optimists), whereas others go through a torrent of negative thoughts throughout the day (the pessimists). The following excerpt from *The Subtleties of the Inimitable Mulla Nasrudin,* a collection of Middle Eastern tales by Idries Shah, demonstrates the point.

I Only Hope I'm Ill

Nasrudin came late among the crowd waiting for the doctor's attentions. He was repeating in a loud voice, over and over again: "I hope I'm very ill, I hope I'm very ill." He so demoralized the other sufferers that they insisted on his going in to see the physician first.

"I only hope I'm very ill!"

"Why?"

"I'd hate to think that anyone who feels like me was really fit and well!" (p. 78)

For obvious reasons, you will want to address the self-talk that is negative. You already feel bad enough, and sustained negative emotions take the joy out of living and contribute to your feelings of helplessness and hopelessness. In addition, as already mentioned, negative self-talk and attitudes can increase disability and dysfunction in chronic pain.

Self-talk is automatic, happens very quickly, and isn't always phrased in complete sentences. For example, let's suppose that you wake up in the morning and open your eyes. You make your first attempt to get out of bed and you become aware of the pain. You might say to yourself: "It's still here. Ugh! I can't stand it any more! When will it go away? I've suffered enough. I'm useless! I'll never get better. This is going to be a miserable day. Life is miserable. I'm miserable. No one cares." If you talk to yourself like this, why *wouldn't* you feel sad or despondent?

However, you should be careful not to confuse the efforts of working on negative thinking with judging thoughts as "good" or "bad." The question is not whether they are good or bad, but whether they are helpful or unhelpful.

We all engage in negative self-talk at one time or another. However, in so doing we often create a reality that just isn't accurate. Much negative self-talk is inaccurate because it distorts events in exaggerated, magnified, all-or-nothing ways that make us feel defeated and helpless. We become victims of the idea that the outside world or external events are responsible for our misery. The self-talk about pain in the "getting out of bed" example is depressing or anxiety-provoking, because it intertwines both realistic and unrealistic descriptions of what's going on. It's true that the pain is still there and you're miserable. However, the other statements are exaggerated, black-and-white assumptions whose accuracy can and should be challenged. You aren't necessarily useless because you have pain; and you really don't know whether the *whole* day will be miserable; and, in any event, what's that got to do with people caring about you?

The power of cognitive work lies in the opportunity it provides you to challenge what you say to yourself. You can reflect on why you feel the way you do and on how you might change that. A passage from *The Pleasantries of the Incredible Mulla Nasrudin,* another of Idries Shah's books, illustrates this:

I Believe You Are Right!

The Mulla was made magistrate. During his first case, the plaintiff argued so persuasively that [Nasrudin] exclaimed: "I believe that you are right!" The clerk of the Court begged him to restrain himself, for the defendant had not been heard yet.

Nasrudin was so carried away by the eloquence of the defendant that he cried out as soon as the man had finished his evidence: "I believe you are right!" The clerk of the court could not allow this.

"Your honor, they cannot *both* be right."

"I believe you are right!" said Nasrudin. (p. 48)

Let's look at an example that illustrates the effects of different interpretations of a situation. Suppose that you are driving to an appointment and get caught in traffic. Imagine yourself responding in two different ways:

Response Set 1

The thoughts: "I can't believe this is happening to me! Where did all these people come from? Don't they know I have an important appointment? I'll never make it on time. This always happens to me. I should have known the traffic would be heavy. I'm so stupid. What a jerk!"

Physical response: Increased blood pressure and heart rate; short, shallow breathing; increased muscle tension . . . in short, the stress response.

Emotional response: Anger, frustration, and guilt.

Response Set 2

The thoughts: "What a drag. This is very unfortunate. My options to get out of this traffic jam are limited because I'm on a bridge. I may be late, but I can't control that right now. I'll use this opportunity to practice some diaphragmatic breathing while I put my favorite Mozart tape in the tape deck. I'll take a mini-vacation!"

Physical response: If anything, a decrease in blood pressure and heart rate; slowed breathing; decreased muscle tension.

Emotional response: Resolution, acceptance, and control.

What are the differences in the two sets of responses? What is it in the nature of the thoughts in Response Set 1 that might predispose you to anger and frustration? Underline the statements in Response Set 1 that are an accurate reflection of the situation. Now consider Response Set 2: How does it differ from Response Set 1? Underline the statements in Response Set 2 that accurately reflect the situation.

Your immediate reaction to all of this may be that you have a right to get agitated and frustrated when bad things happen. You certainly do! But we are talking about choices. If getting aggravated and agitated is your preferred mode of operation, go right ahead. If, however, you find that negative emotional states increase your emotional distress and your physical pain, then read on.

Irrational and Distorted Thoughts

Where do these "wild and crazy" thoughts come from? Why are they sometimes such distortions of what is really going on? Modern psychology and research on consciousness are only now beginning to appreciate the potential of the mind and the need for all of us to understand how and why we think the way we do.

The following observations (see "Supplementary Reading") may stimulate you to begin your own journey toward greater awareness of your thinking processes:

- Our cultural beliefs and vocabulary influence what we perceive of the world around us (Edward Hall and Robert Cialdini).
- Our predisposition for short-term planning leaves us vulnerable to long-term consequences (Robert Ornstein).
- Gender, as well as culture, influences our interpersonal communication (Deborah Tannen).

A good place to start is to identify the content of the assumptions and beliefs that lie behind your self-talk. Psychologists and other thinkers have made several attempts at identifying the sources of negative thoughts, and these ideas are not necessarily new.

Men are disturbed not by things which happen, but by the opinions about the things. . . . When we are impeded or disturbed or grieved, let us never blame others, but ourselves, that is our opinion. It is the act of an ill-instructed man to blame others for his bad condition; it is the act of one who has begun to be instructed, to lay the blame on himself; and of one whose instruction is completed, neither to blame another, nor himself. (Epictetus, circa A.D. 55–135, *The Encheiridion*)

Ellis's Irrational Beliefs

One psychologist, Albert Ellis, has developed a model for challenging exaggerated thoughts and replacing them with more realistic ones. This model is called "rational–emotive therapy"; its basic premise is that much of our suffering comes from the irrational ways we perceive the world. The exaggerated, self-defeating thoughts we engage in lead to pessimism and ineffectual behaviors and limit our possibilities. Here is a list of Ellis's ten "irrational beliefs" (from Ellis; see "Supplementary Reading"). I like to call them "the assumptions and beliefs that get us into trouble."

1. It is an absolute necessity for an adult to have love and approval from peers, family, and friends.
2. You must be unfailingly competent and almost perfect in all you undertake.
3. Certain people are evil, wicked, and villainous and should be punished.
4. It is horrible when people and things are not the way you would like them to be.
5. External events cause most human misery—people simply react as events trigger their emotions.

6. You should feel fear or anxiety about anything that is unknown, uncertain, or potentially dangerous.
7. It is easier to avoid than to face life's difficulties and responsibilities.
8. You need something other or stronger or greater than yourself to rely on.
9. The past has a lot to do with determining the present.
10. Happiness can be achieved by inaction, passivity, and endless leisure.

These beliefs are not *necessarily* irrational or crazy. That is, they are not absolutely untrue under all circumstances. But they are certainly irrational if you believe in them unwaveringly—if you believe that they are absolutely true under all circumstances and allow them to govern your thoughts and behaviors accordingly. For example, making mistakes does feel horrible, but it is also part of being human. The lesson is to learn from them.

The Nature of "Truth"

Your first response after reading the list of Ellis's irrational beliefs may be this: "But how can these be irrational? They are all true!" If so, take a moment to think about the nature of "truth."

I'll never forget talking to a group of patients one time about how they felt when someone passed them in the breakdown lane while they were sitting in a traffic jam on a major beltway around Boston. The condemnations poured out: "They have no right to do that." "They're creeps." "Where are the police when you need them?" I then asked how many had *never* driven in the breakdown lane on that road. No one raised his or her hand.

We get caught up in the "truth" sometimes, but whose "truth" are we talking about? A passage from a third Idries Shah collection, *The Exploits of the Incomparable Mulla Nasrudin,* illustrates that this can be a tricky question:

How Nasrudin Created Truth

"Laws as such do not make people better," said Nasrudin to the King. "They must practice certain things in order to become attuned to inner truth. This *form* of truth resembles apparent truth only slightly."

The King decided that he could, and would, make people observe the truth. He could make them practice truthfulness.

His city was entered by a bridge. On this he built a gallows. The following day, when the gates were opened at dawn, the Captain of the Guard was stationed with a squad of troops to examine all who entered.

An announcement was made: "Everyone will be questioned. If he tells the truth, he will be allowed to enter. If he lies, he will be hanged."

Nasrudin stepped forward.

"Where are you going?"

"I am on my way," said Nasrudin slowly, "to be hanged."

"We don't believe you!"

"Very well, if I have told a lie, hang me!"

"But if we hang you for lying, we will have made what you said come true!"

"That's right; now you know what the truth is—YOUR truth!" (p. 7)

Burns's 10 Types of Cognitive Distortions

Another model for classifying negative self-talk comes from David Burns, a psychiatrist whose writings on cognitive techniques have been instrumental in bringing these powerful mind tools to a wider public. He found 10 common cognitive distortions that can contribute to negative emotions. They also fuel catastrophic thinking patterns that are particularly disabling. Read the following and see if you can identify ones that are familiar to you:

1. *All-or-nothing thinking.* This refers to the tendency to evaluate personal qualities or situations in extreme, black-or-white categories. For example, before you developed chronic pain, you used to play baseball on the weekends. Now you find yourself thinking, "If I can't play baseball, I can't enjoy the sport anymore."

   There is an apparent advantage to thinking in black-and-white, all-or-nothing terms. It is more predictable and creates the feeling that there is order in the world around you. This, in turn, should give you an edge to controlling your world. Unfortunately, it doesn't work that way. Uncertainty is all that we have. Living comfortably with uncertainty is possible, but it takes time to master. The skills you are about to learn will help.

2. *Overgeneralization.* This refers to the tendency to see a single negative event as a never-ending pattern of defeat. If you wake up in more pain, you might respond, "I'll never be able to enjoy anything anymore." Misery does love company, but globalizing misfortune in this way creates an exaggerated sense of rejection and loneliness.

3. *Mental filtering.* This refers to the tendency to dwell exclusively on a single negative event and thus to perceive the whole situation as negative. For example, you are preparing lunch for some friends and discover that you do not have an essential ingredient to make a dish you were planning to include. All you can think about is how the whole lunch will be ruined. It gives you indigestion.

4. *Disqualifying the positive.* This refers to the tendency to take neutral or even positive experiences and turn them into negative ones. For example, a friend comes over to visit and tells you that you look great. Your immediate thought is this: "I don't feel great. She doesn't understand." Maybe not, but try a simple "thank you" first before you check it out. Maybe you don't look as bad as you feel!

5. *Jumping to conclusions.* This refers specifically to jumping to a negative conclusion that is not justified by the facts of the situation. Two types of jumping to conclusions are mind reading and fortune telling.

   A. *Mind reading.* You assume you know why someone else does what he or she does, and you don't bother to check it out. For example, you pass a coworker in the hallway and say "Hi!" He doesn't respond. You think, "He must be upset with me. What did I do wrong?" When you check it out, you find that the coworker was preoccupied about a sick child he had just left at home.

B. *Fortune telling.* You "know" that things will turn out badly. Given your bad luck, you predict it is an established fact. For example, you wake up with a headache. You say, "Now my whole day is ruined. I had so much to do and I'll never get it all done."

6. *Magnification and minification.* In magnification, you exaggerate the importance of a negative event or mistake. If, for example, you experience a flare-up in your pain, you find yourself saying, "I can't stand this! I can't take this any more!" As a matter of fact, however, you can. You may not want to, and that's okay, but you can take it. In minification, conversely, you take positive personal qualities or events and deny them their importance. For example, a family member comments on how nice it is to see you at a family outing, and you reply, " A lot of good it does if I can't participate in the activities."

7. *Emotional reasoning.* This refers to taking your emotions as evidence for the truth. If you *feel* that something is right, then it must be true. For example, you find yourself thinking, "I feel useless. [Therefore] I *am* useless."

8. *Labeling.* This refers specifically to identifying a mistake or negative quality and then describing an entire situation or individual in terms of that quality. For example, instead of seeing yourself as an individual who has a pain problem, you find yourself saying, "I'm defective, imperfect, and without any redeemable qualities."

9. *Personalization.* This refers to taking responsibility for a negative event even when the circumstances are beyond your control. For example, you and your spouse go out to eat at a fancy restaurant, but the service and food are poor. You find yourself feeling responsible for making a bad choice and "ruining" your evening together.

10. *"Should" statements.* These are attempts to motivate (or browbeat) yourself by saying things like "I should know better," "I should go there," or "I must do that." Such statements set you up for feeling resentful and pressured. They also imply that you are complying with an external authority.

Old "Tapes"

The irrational beliefs and cognitive distortions described above are old "tapes" that we play from our early experiences as children. They reflect the observed responses of our families, our teachers, and the society in which we develop. Loretta Laroche, a comedian who teaches these principles through humor, conjures up a powerful image of a big yellow school bus that each person drives through life. Various people get on and off, but some have a lifetime ticket. They may include parents, teachers, ex-lovers, friends, and mentors, both alive and dead. There's always someone who thinks he or she knows the best way of getting where you're going, and sometimes that person will be found in the driver's seat. But this is your opportunity to decide who's really driving your bus. To return to the "tapes" metaphor, it's your opportunity to edit your old tapes and make some new ones.

There are different kinds of tapes, with different recurring themes. For example, you either assume all the responsibility or none of it ("The pain is all my fault" or "The pain is all your fault"). Or you expect a consistency in the world that doesn't exist ("If I'm good, bad things won't happen to me"). Or perhaps you feel that if you think negatively, it will ward off bad fortune ("I'm feeling better this morning, but if I tell anyone the pain might get worse"). Thinking in restricted, unconscious patterns (the old tapes) often robs you of the flexibility needed to cope with the ever-changing world and your personal problems.

Monitoring Self-Talk (Automatic Thoughts)

An Exercise Format

Using the exercise format described here each time you find yourself feeling sad, frustrated, or anxious will allow you to begin to act, rather than react, toward events occurring around you. Again, it is not the intention of this exercise in particular or this chapter in general to judge the "goodness" or "badness" of negative thinking. The problem with thinking negatively for extended periods is simply that it is not helpful for problem solving and for responding effectively to what's going on around you.

The following example illustrates what this exercise covers:

You wake up with increased pain on a day you had planned to visit a friend. (*Situation*)

What would you find yourself thinking? (*Automatic thoughts*) _____

How would you feel physically? (*Physical response*) _____

How would you feel emotionally? (*Emotional response*) _____

What are the irrational beliefs or cognitive distortions you would be engaged in? Refer to the previous pages where these are listed. (*Cognitive distortions*) _____

What is really going on and what action can you take? (*Changed thought*, to be discussed later) _____

At the back of the book, there is a "Daily Record of Automatic Thoughts (Self-Talk)" worksheet that you can copy and carry with you to capture and record your automatic thoughts and other responses to stressful events in just this manner. You can't always count on memory, because the emotional arousal and negative cognitive responses will most likely diminish as time passes. You may be aware only of physical symptoms, such as muscle tension or palpitations, and not the emotions or thoughts. By writing down as much as you can about the situation and your physical sensations, you will be able to recapture the emotions and thoughts. Slowly, with time and practice, you will be able to change these negative responses as they occur. Remember, too, that this exercise can be used to explore your negative emotions and cognitions about anything, not just your pain.

Working with Anger

Anger is a powerful emotion. It is particularly important to control because of its potential health risks (heart disease, substance abuse) and the risk of social damage that can be done under its influence (road rage, sexual and physical abuse). Many people experience anger as a reaction to frustration or hurt. When someone or something has hurt you, the fight, instead of flight, reaction may be triggered. This can be difficult to control because it is associated with a major adrenalin rush. Much of the work with self-talk has to do with agreeing to change the way you respond to events. But being angry can make such changes difficult. Anger is associated with blaming the outside world in general or with specific events or people whom you feel have caused your problem. That attitude can be a problem if you can't give it its proper place.

For many people giving up their anger feels as though they are giving up or giving in to guilt for a pain problem that may clearly not have been their fault. Assigning responsibility for an injury—the driver ran the red light and hit my car—can bring about resolution or closure of wrongdoing. However, holding on to the anger about the wrongdoing contributes to feelings of victimization, depression, and anxiety. Specific exercises to help assess and control anger can be very helpful. You've already started doing many of them. They include relaxation techniques to help buy time between the event and emotional response, physical exercise that helps check the stress effects of anger, the thinking skills we've started to address in this chapter, and journaling and communication skills that are described later. We discuss anger more fully in the next chapter. Other resources for anger management can be found in "Supplementary Reading."

"Why Me?"

Sometimes you may find yourself saying, "Why did this happen to me? When will it end? Why me? Why? Why? Why?" These questions can overwhelm you with anxiety, because they may give you an unrealistic sense that you *should* be able to answer the questions. Asking such questions may also give you the illusion that the problems behind them are being explored and are about to be solved. In fact, however, no definite answers to such questions are possible.

Instead, you need to look at the assumptions behind the questions. For example, do you feel that there is a reason for everything and that you should know it? Do you have a secret fear that anyone who feels this horrible must have done something pretty bad? If you were told that your pain would end in exactly six years and two months, would you be able to live comfortably now? Once you have identified these assumptions, compare them with the lists of irrational beliefs and cognitive distortions provided earlier. Which ones do your assumptions contain?

The "Why?" questions are not to be confused with those associated with the search for meaning in all our lives. Meaning won't be found in an endless litany of "Why me?"; such questions are, in the end, just another form of negative thinking.

Changing Your Thoughts

> The greatest revolution of our time is the knowledge that human beings, by changing the inner attitudes of their minds, can transform the outer aspects of their lives.
>
> —*William James*

You can begin changing your self-talk by using one of three techniques.

Technique 1: Challenging Self-Talk (Automatic Thoughts)

In this first technique, you challenge the reality of your self-talk as follows: First, identify or capture the negative, automatic thoughts. Next, examine the captured thoughts for the distortions, irrational beliefs, and self-defeating attitudes that may have caused you to think and feel this way. With this groundwork in place, you can then challenge the accuracy of the thoughts. Often, after the thoughts are challenged, the emotional response disappears. At other times, describing the reality of the situation to yourself will help you alter the feeling.

For example, is it true that if you have chronic pain, you're defective and imperfect? By now, I would hope that you can respond with a loud "No!" What *is* true is this: You have a chronic problem that alters the way you engage in activities. The statement "I'm defective" is a gross exaggeration of the "labeling" kind (number 8 in Burns's list of cognitive distortions). Recognizing this, you may now be able to say something like the following to yourself: "Being in pain curtails my activities, but it does not reflect on my character, " or "I have found that by pacing my activities I can still accomplish things and I can feel good about myself, because I have demonstrated the courage to rise above my disability." How does that feel?

Be careful about one thing, however. This changing of the thoughts does *not* mean substituting a positive but inaccurate, exaggerated statement for a negative one—for example, awakening in pain and saying, "This is a wonderful experience" instead of "My whole day is ruined." You will know when you hit on the right statement because you will feel better, relieved, less anxious, or less sad.

Using Technique 1, how might you alter your response to your waking up with increased pain on a day you had made plans to visit a friend? Write your new self-talk here.

_____

_____

_____

Technique 2: Clarifying the Problem and What You Can Do

Here is a second way to change your self-talk. It helps to clarify the real problem after the negative self-talk has been identified. It also serves to give you an idea of where you have the control or power in a seemingly impossible situation. Here is an example:

State the problem: *I am awakening in pain.*

State why it's a problem: *Because I had plans to visit a friend today.*

Identify:

What can you do?   *I will see how I feel after taking a hot shower, an RR technique, and taking two aspirin.*

What do you need?   *I can ask that my friend come here, or that we meet somewhere closer. Or I can visit her another time. This happens. It is usually self-limited. I know what I can do to take care of myself.*

How do you feel?   *Sad, but in control.*

Technique 3: The Vertical Arrow or "So What?" Technique

Sometimes you may have trouble seeing where the problem is with your self-talk. It just seems so accurate, and you feel even more miserable. In these situations, a third way to look at changing your thoughts is the Vertical Arrow Technique, designed by David Burns (see "Supplementary Reading"). In this technique, you take a different approach to your negative thoughts. You begin by buying into the negative self-talk and asking yourself, "If what I'm saying to myself is true, then why does it upset me?" "So what?" or "What's the worst that could happen?" You then write out your responses to these questions and imagine an arrow—or actually draw one—extending down from what you have written.

Next, you ask yourself the same questions, but this time about the response that you just wrote down. You then write down another set of responses, then another arrow, and ask yourself the questions again. You continue until you have uncovered all of the cognitive distortions, irrational beliefs, fears, and assumptions that were hidden beneath the original thought that you were examining. Here is an example:

You wake up in pain. You say, "I'm so useless." First you ask yourself, "If this is true, why does it upset me?" "So what?" or "What's the worst that could happen?"

↓

You may respond, "I can never do anything anybody wants me to do." Ask yourself again, "If this is true, why does it upset me?" "So what?" (The arrow now represents the questions.)

↓

You may respond "Now my friend will hate me because I'm unreliable." Ask yourself, "So what?"

↓

You reply, "Soon I'll have no friends." Ask yourself, "So what?"

↓

You reply, "I'm afraid of being alone." Ask yourself, "So what?"

↓

You reply, "Being alone is the worst thing that can happen to me."

And so on. In the example above, the underlying fear of being alone can make any situation that isolates you the source of depression and panic. Once you know where the panic is coming from, you can take steps to cope with the loneliness.

The completion of the Dysfunctional Attitude Scale (DAS) (unfortunate name but helpful tool), presented at the end of this chapter, can help you identify the beliefs and distortions of thinking that make you vulnerable to daily stresses. My colleagues and I have found the DAS very helpful in identifying the roots of some of the troubling expectations and assumptions people harbor (often unknowingly, until they are challenged). For example, if you score lowest in Perfectionism and Achievement on the DAS, you may find that a majority of your negative feelings recorded during a week were generated during scenarios challenging your beliefs that you must achieve perfectly all the time (e.g., "If I can't work, I don't deserve to do anything fun"; "If I make a mistake, I'm stupid and inadequate"; "I'm a terrible father if I can't play baseball with my kids"). Challenging such inflexible assumptions and expectations is part of getting to drive your own yellow school bus or make your own tapes (to borrow two metaphors used earlier in this chapter).

The Narrative Repair

"The narrative repair" is the name given to the technique of writing about stressful or traumatic events. Keeping diaries or journals is certainly not new, but research into the powerful healing effects of putting words down on paper is. Research performed by James Pennebaker, described in his book *Opening Up: The Healing Power of Expressing Emotions* (see "Supplementary Reading"), and others has demonstrated that writing about your stresses and traumas can be therapeutic. Furthermore, there appears to be an evolving process as an individual continues to write, the narrative repair, that is associated with bringing coherence (making sense) or meaning to the traumatic experience. Bringing meaning to the pain experience can be an important step to healing and decreasing long-term disability. Writing that is self-reflective (not self-absorbed or intellectual) will be the most therapeutic. It is not meant to be another form of complaining or a diversion from acting on a problem.

Changing Self-Talk Practice

These techniques will not make everything that happens to you stressless. However, they can allow you to identify your choices and control your responses to life's daily hassles and major challenges. You will feel differently when you can describe what is going on and determine your options. David Burns's books are highly recommended for further work in this area (see "Supplementary Reading").

Try practicing with all three of the techniques presented here. Changing how you feel by changing what you say to yourself may be such an unusual idea that you will need practice to become skilled at it. Most likely, in the beginning, the best you can do will be to look at your thoughts after the fact. Eventually, however, you will be able to start questioning as soon as you start hearing your inner chatter. You will know when you have captured the thoughts that created your negative emotions, because just by reading them you will recreate the emotions. But beware of the "Why me?" questions. Go beyond to the assumptions or expectations that underlie such questions. You will know when you've hit upon an adequate change of a thought, because you will feel better and more in control.

Now let's take a look at what happened to Joan (see the quote at the beginning of the chapter). By the end of the program, her thinking had undergone a transformation. The following is the beginning of a poem she wrote, based on a dream she had during the program:

A friend showed me a grey cement urn, the size of a well. It opened slightly.

Inside were limbs, arms, and legs floating in a thin, dark liquid.

A man dove to the bottom and brought my body to the surface. It was not dead, only half dead—kept alive somehow by a mask and snorkel.

I was afraid to look at it, but I did—

When I saw that it was me, I turned to my friend and husband and said with utter joy: "I'm so glad to be living."

I watched the man lift my body from the urn and begin to walk with it. My body slowly began to come to life.

The man led my body onto a boat where a crowd was gathered to watch. The two walked through the middle of the crowd of people.

As they did so, my body was transformed. It became filled with light and covered by white flowing garments. The head became covered with long, golden hair.

At the bow of the boat, my body sailed off into the sky and the crowd of people cheered.

I thought to myself as I watched: "I am beautiful!"

The Role of Psychology in Chronic Pain

There has been a great deal of debate in medicine about whether or not chronic pain is simply the physical manifestation of psychological trauma, depression, or hysteria. Many believe that chronic pain has a psychological or psychosomatic cause. The psychological theories of the origins of chronic pain have gained popularity in part because of the separation of mind and body in the discipline of medicine. In addition, ignorance of the mechanisms responsible for chronic pain has contributed to the idea that what can't be seen must be "psychological."

Many doctors emphasize either the body or the mind in their therapies. A body doctor rarely explores the emotional or psychological manifestations of living in pain, and a mind doctor seldom if ever physically examines a patient. Yet, as I listen to chronic pain patients describe what their physical, emotional, and social limitations are, it is very clear to me that the mind *and* body are intimately involved in the experience of chronic pain. It is important to make psychological diagnoses so that appropriate treatment can be prescribed; however, there may be too much psychological labeling of chronic pain patients who do not get better. This only serves to increase everyone's frustration and devalues the patients' experience; it does not clarify therapeutic approaches. Let's explore some of the psychological labels that are commonly used in chronic pain.

Common Psychological Labels in Chronic Pain

Depression

In the absence of pain, feeling sad or worthless and having trouble sleeping or eating may lead to a diagnosis of depression. But in a person experiencing pain, these common symptoms can be indicative of the struggle to live with the pain, which can be quite disruptive. The treatment of an individual with chronic pain may include antidepressants but should be a part of a comprehensive treatment plan.

Depressed patients also complain of bodily aches and pains. The difference is that the pain complaints usually go away with satisfactory treatment of the depression. In chronic pain, the pain doesn't go away with the treatment of the depression, although the pain *experience* may improve.

Hysteria

Many women patients with chronic pain are incorrectly labeled as "hysterical," simply because they are female and have unexplained pain complaints. "Hysteria" is a term with great historical interest. In medical writings as recently as the last century, the womb (in Greek, *hystera*) was considered to be the source of many a female problem, making a woman prone to moodiness, fickleness, irritability, and multiple physical complaints. These "abnormal," "hysterical" behaviors contrasted with the expected calm, rational social behavior of the "normal" (i.e., male) population.

Hysteria as a mental illness was described as early as the 16th century. Again, it was described as occurring primarily in women (though men were occasionally described as experiencing the illness as well). Sigmund Freud influenced the current psychiatric understanding of hysteria. He wrote extensively about his speculations concerning the cause and treatment of a mysterious loss of physical function involving almost any part of the body and associated with psychological traumas (usually involving sexual conflict).

The hysterical patients were also characterized by a particular emotional response called *la belle indifference*. That is, they did not seem to care about their loss of function, such as their inability to speak or walk. Typically, patients with chronic pain care very much about their loss of function.

Given either the historically sexist meaning or the specific psychiatric condition described by Freud, the use of the term "hysterical" to describe the observations of chronic pain in an anxious or frightened female (or male) patient does not appear to be appropriate or accurate, even if the response is thought to be an exaggerated one. Nor does the fact that X-ray or laboratory findings cannot delineate the source or cause of chronic pain in a patient justify a diagnosis of hysteria or the labeling of pain behaviors as "hysterical." We would do better to observe that pain behaviors are manifestations of suffering that occur in a woman *or* man with chronic pain. We also need to realize that "appropriate behaviors" are culturally and socially determined and as such are subject to interpretation and bias.

Hypochondriasis

Some individuals are intensely preoccupied and worried about their health. They are sensitive to the physical sensations that arise from the normal functioning of their bodies and may become alarmed if they become aware of such things as their own normal heartbeat. They are rarely reassured, or at best only temporarily reassured, by examinations or testing by their doctors. Such individuals are referred to as "hypochondriacs."

From this book's previous discussions about the experience of chronic pain and the lack of a clear-cut cause in many cases, it is easy to see how the label of "hypochondriacs" might be misapplied to chronic pain patients. Patients with pain syndromes such as fibromyalgia (see Appendix A)—in which the pain is ill defined, diffuse, intermittent, and migratory, with no specific diagnostic laboratory confirmation—have reported such misunderstandings. In such cases, it is essential that a careful history and examination be performed. The pattern of symptoms, the presence of the tender points, and the absence of positive results for rheumatoid arthritis or lupus on laboratory tests can help make the diagnosis of fibromyalgia. In addition, the willingness of patients with fibromyalgia to be active participants in their pain management, working in partnership with their health care providers, demonstrates a healthy coping response. This would be an unlikely response in patients suffering from hypochondriasis.

Malingering

There appears to be considerable paranoia on the part of many insurance companies and physicians about chronic pain sufferers' being "malingerers"—people who only pretend to be ill. Such paranoia generates blame and distrust between health care providers and patients. This state of affairs is probably due in part to the "who's to blame," litigious atmosphere in which medicine is currently practiced. It's hard enough for physicians and other care providers to make accurate diagnoses and treat symptoms, without also wondering whether the symptoms being reported are "real." The lack of clearly defined explanations for chronic pain in humans also causes considerable confusion on the part of practitioners about the reality of chronic pain. Further misunderstanding is created by a physician's perception that a patient has somehow failed in or has sabotaged "usually successful" therapy and by a patient's corresponding perception that the physician has failed to deliver relief from pain and suffering.

If a health care provider and a patient in pain are to have a successful therapeutic relationship, their mutual blame and distrust must be put aside. These feelings must be replaced with the realization that the experience of chronic pain is real, not imaginary or invented. Chronic pain is not a curable problem for many patients, but the symptoms can be reduced. Furthermore, chronic pain is not a matter of failure to respond on a patient's part or failure to provide effective treatment on a physician's part.

As discussed in Chapter 2, chronic pain is a complex experience of a warning system gone awry. A patient's search for the meaning of the pain can lead him or her to focus on finding someone to blame, particularly when pain occurs after an accident. Although the prospect of being compensated as a result of a legal action or worker's compensation injury may influence the experience of pain, it does not appear to create pain in the majority of individuals. As is discussed later, many a compensation scenario is associated with anger and frustration, which can interfere with healing and can worsen the pain experience. When the legal system, worker's compensation, or a disability insurer becomes involved in an individual's case, there is often a lengthening of the normal grieving process and a delay in coming to acceptance of the chronic pain condition. This delay is not malingering, however.

In short, patients are responsible for clearly and accurately reporting their pain experience; physicians are responsible for thorough evaluation and treatment; and external systems need to provide compensation in a timely and just manner.

Posttraumatic Stress Disorder

Considerable attention is currently being given to the physical and psychological manifestations of posttraumatic stress disorder (PTSD). Some theorists believe that certain types of chronic pain (e.g., headaches, abdominal pain, and pelvic pain) are really the psychological manifestations of some sexual or physical abuse that occurred years before.

Another explanation, however, may be that for those with chronic pain *and* an experience of significant physical or emotional trauma, having chronic pain *feels* like being abused again. Feelings of anxiety, vulnerability, lack of control, and not being believed can be experienced both by patients in pain and by people with PTSD. It is therefore possible for persons who have been abused or experienced significant trauma *and* who have chronic pain to experience a magnification of their pain, both emotionally and physically. The PTSD may not cause the pain in these circumstances, but it may compound the experience of physical pain because of the similar qualities of these two emotion-laden experiences. To put it another way, the psychological distress of PTSD needs treating, and so does the physical pain.

It is important, however, to explore for the presence of PTSD before multiple surgical or medical procedures are performed. For example, in persistent pelvic pain, the pain

distress may not reach a magnitude that would precipitate or encourage surgical intervention if such coexisting factors as PTSD are treated as well. The relationship between
PTSD and pain is an important connection to be explored, because the healing must take
place at multiple levels—in the memories of the mind *and* the body.

Summary

- We know that certain ways of thinking are commonly associated with disability in
  chronic pain and poor coping in stressful times, for example, catastrophizing, denial, avoidance, and wishful thinking.
- Automatic thoughts or self-talk can affect the way you feel. Furthermore, if you
  can alter or change your negative self-talk, you can actually change how you feel.
- Our cultural beliefs and vocabulary influence how we perceive the world around
  us; our predisposition for short-term planning leaves us vulnerable to long-term
  consequences; and gender, as well as culture, influences our interpersonal communication.
- Albert Ellis has developed a method called "rational–emotive therapy" to challenge irrational beliefs and replace them with more realistic ones.
- David Burns has developed another method for approaching negative self-talk. He
  has identified 10 categories of "cognitive distortions" that can lead to negative
  emotional states.
- Monitoring your self-talk and physical/emotional responses to stressful situations
  will enable you to evaluate and begin to change these responses. Anger and
  thoughts of "Why me?" require particularly careful examination.
- Changing thoughts associated with negative emotional states allows you to identify your options and gain greater control over your responses to life's difficulties.
  Three techniques are presented:

  - Challenging the reality of your self-talk
  - Clarifying the problem and developing an action plan
  - The Vertical Arrow ("So What?") Technique for those more difficult-to-reach
    agendas

- Psychological labels for chronic pain patients are of benefit when such labels are
  used as a means of understanding the process and formulating a treatment plan.

Exploration Tasks

1. Using the "Daily Record of Automatic Thoughts (Self-Talk)":

    Keep track of what you are thinking whenever you experience a negative emotional
    state (sadness, anxiety, fear, or jealousy) or whenever you are feeling increased

Sample Daily Record of Automatic Thoughts (Self-Talk)

Date	Situation	Automatic thoughts	Physical response	Emotional response	Cognitive distortion	Changed thought
Example: 1/02/00	*Pain flare-up*	*Can't take this.* *I can't do anything.*	↑ *tension* *crying*	*Helpless* *Frustrated*	*All or nothing* *Magnification*	1. *Pain increases are scary.* 2. *I've been through this before.* 3. *I have tools I can apply to get through this.* 4. *This is what I'll do . . .*

Adapted from Aaron T. Beck et al., *Cognitive Therapy of Depression* (New York: Guilford Press, 1979). Copyright 1979 by Aaron T. Beck, A. John Rush, Brian F. Shaw, and Gary Emery. Adapted by permission.

physical tension or pain. (You have automatic thoughts with positive emotional states, too, but clearly you don't need to work on changing those emotional states.) Copy and use the "Daily Record of Automatic Thoughts (Self-Talk)" provided at the end of this book.

- First identify and record the event or situation associated with negative (sadness, self-defeated, anxious) emotions. For example: *Pain flare-up*.
- Write down your thoughts (capturing them on paper): *"I can't take it anymore."*
- Write down the physical symptoms you experience at these stressful times: *"Muscle tension, heartburn."*
- Write down the emotional response: *"Out of control, helpless."*
- Write down the distortion, the belief behind the thoughts: *"If I can't take it someone else will [wishful thinking]. It's beyond my control and there is nothing I can do to help myself [all-or-nothing thinking, catastrophic thinking]."*
- Using one of the three techniques, see if you can challenge the distortions and thoughts that are unrealistic. Come up with more realistic, action-oriented thoughts and phrases: *"The reality is that I can take it and have. I don't have to like it. I have many things I can do to manage my pain flare-up."*

2. Certain techniques can facilitate identifying, capturing, and changing your self-talk.

   A. The regular practice of RR techniques (see Chapter 3) does facilitate this self-observation. If you have not been practicing a daily RR technique, you may have more difficulties capturing these quick thoughts and may wish to consider increasing your commitment to daily RR practice.

   B. Journaling can help you identify the automatic thoughts that you may have trouble observing, identifying, or admitting. The most common problem when people begin to start monitoring their self-talk is that they do not go beyond describing their mood. They do not explore the thoughts that are responsible for the mood.

They go immediately to problem solving. Although problem solving is where we want to go with these exercises, you may not be ready yet. Unless you want to be always a victim, you need first to see what drives these ever-present self-defeating thoughts. That means identifying the thoughts that make you sad, angry, or anxious and the beliefs that are driving them—fear of losing control, not being loved, being used by others, and so forth. Journaling is a way of taking the time to capture the thoughts, all of them, and explore the assumptions behind them. Usually people find that they have a few common distortions that run through most of their self-talk. Taking the time to reflect on these common scenarios will allow you to gain more mastery over them. Write about a stressful event for 10–20 minutes, letting whatever comes up flow out onto the paper (or if this is difficult because of your particular site of pain, use a tape recorder). You do not have to share it with anyone. See what comes up. What are the familiar themes? Phrases? Do not be surprised if you feel the emotion more intensely. You are getting to the roots of your despair. Only after you get it all out on paper do you start working on the changing of the self-statements, challenging the reality of what you have said and identifying the distortions. If anger is a dominant theme, try the next exercise.

3. Anger, as I pointed out before, is a challenge. There are many reasons people become angry; this exercise deals with only a few of them. People injured by someone else in an accident or at work often feel angry at the other person. A *threat*, apparent or real, at the "hands of others" can be quite distressful. Being a victim feels awful. But why? Can you capture or identify why you feel angry? (Substituting the word "hurt" or "frustration" for "anger" may be easier for some people to identify with.) For example: *"I feel angry (hurt, frustrated) because that person was careless when he ran the red light and could have killed me!"*

_____

_____

_____

Can you identify how the other person may think from *his or her* point of view? *"It was a mistake, I didn't mean to, I shouldn't have been talking on the cell phone, it was stupid."*

_____

_____

_____

When you think about the threatening incident, what does your body do in response to the angry thoughts? (*breath holding, increased muscle tension, increased blood pressure*)

_____

_____

_____

When you think about the incident from the other person's viewpoint, how does your body respond?

_____

_____

_____

What are the advantages *to you* of staying angry? What might be the disadvantages?

_____

_____

_____

Can you identify ways to suffer less physically because of your anger? (*relaxation techniques, breathing through the tension while thinking of your anger*)

_____

_____

_____

Can you identify ways to suffer less emotionally because of your anger? (*consider meditation; look to the future for what I can do, not to the past for what I've lost*)

_____

_____

_____

4. Complete the Dysfunctional Attitude Scale (DAS) provided at the end of this chapter. After you identify the categories in which you scored the lowest (the minus numbers or the lowest positive numbers), look at the five questions composing each category and identify the irrational beliefs or cognitive distortions associated with them. Use this information to help challenge some of the irrational self-talk you engage in from time to time and to identify patterns in various events that disrupt your peace of mind. You may feel upset by what you find out, but remember that the truth can set you free.

5. Making Use of the Dysfunctional Attitude Scale

When you find yourself reacting to your pain or life events in a negative way with frustration, feelings of defeat, giving up, giving in . . .

A. STOP, TAKE A DEEP BREATH.

B. Ask yourself, "What is going on here? Are these my old tapes or assumptions playing out here?"

C. "Where do I have control here? What can I do?"

D. PRACTICE, PRACTICE, PRACTICE.

6. Write out a goal that you want to accomplish related to this chapter. As always, make sure your goal is a behavioral task that you can measure in terms of the steps *you* will take to accomplish it. Here is an example:

Goal: *Keep track of my automatic thoughts when I become aware that I am depressed or anxious.*

Steps to take to reach that goal:

A. *Copy the chart at the back of the book and carry it in my pocket.*

B. *If I can't capture the automatic thoughts, I'll use the writing exercise to write about each incident and see what comes up.*

C. *After completing the DAS, I will examine the nature of the situations that were associated with the depression or anxiety and see if they match any of my self-defeating attitudes by the DAS.*

Now it's your turn.

Goal: _____

Steps to take to reach that goal:

A. _____

B. _____

C. _____

D. _____

In addition, list contingency plans. That is, identify what obstacles might get in the way of your accomplishing this goal. What solutions can you devise to work toward insuring the success of this goal?

	Obstacles	**Solutions**
A.	_____	_____
B.	_____	_____
C.	_____	_____
D.	_____	_____

Supplementary Reading

The following books provide additional ideas and observations regarding how and why we think the way we do:

David Burns, *The Feeling Good Handbook* (New York: Plume, 1999).
David Burns, *Ten Days to Self-Esteem* (New York: Quill/William Morrow, 1999).
Robert Cialdini, *Influence: The Psychology of Persuasion* (New York: Quill/William Morrow, 1993).

Albert Ellis, *How to Make Yourself Happy and Remarkably Less Disturbable* (Manassas Park, VA: Impact Publications, 1999).

Edward T. Hall, *Beyond Culture* (New York: Anchor, 1977).

Matthew McKay and Peter Rogers, *The Anger Control Workbook* (Oakland, CA: New Harbinger Publications, 2000).

Robert Ornstein, *Evolution of Consciousness* (New York: Touchstone, 1992).

Robert Ornstein, *The Psychology of Consciousness* (New York: Penguin Books, 1986).

James Pennebaker, *Opening Up: The Healing Power of Expressing Emotions* (New York: Guilford Press, 1997).

Martin Seligman, *Learned Optimism* (New York: Pocket Books, 1998).

Idries Shah, *The Pleasantries of the Incredible Mulla Nasrudin* (London: Octagon Press, 1983).

Idries Shah, *Reflections* (London: Octagon Press, 1983).

Idries Shah, *The Subtleties of the Inimitable Mulla Nasrudin* and *The Exploits of the Incomparable Mulla Nasrudin* (London: Octagon Press, 1989).

Deborah Tannen, *You Just Don't Understand: Women and Men in Conversation* (New York: Ballantine Books, 1991).

Hendria Weisinger, *Dr. Weisinger's Anger Workout Book* (New York: Quill, 1985).

Denise Winn, *The Manipulated Mind: Brainwashing, Conditioning and Manipulation* (Los Altos, CA: Malor Books, 2000).

Dysfunctional Attitude Scale (DAS)

Instructions

As you fill out the questionnaire, indicate how much you agree or disagree with each attitude. When you are finished, an answer key will let you score your answers and generate a profile of your personal values systems. This will show your areas of psychological strength and vulnerability.

Answering the test is quite simple. After each of the 35 attitudes, put a check in the column that represents your estimate of how you think *most* of the time. Be sure to choose only one answer for each attitude. Because we are all different, there is no "right" or "wrong" answer to any statement. To decide whether a given attitude is typical of your own philosophy, recall how you look at things most of the time.

Statement	Agree strongly	Agree slightly	Neutral	Disagree slightly	Disagree very much
1. Criticism will obviously upset the person who receives the criticism.	____	____	____	____	____
2. It is best to give up my own interests in order to please other people.	____	____	____	____	____
3. I need other people's approval in order to be happy.	____	____	____	____	____
4. If someone important to me expects me to do something, then I really should do it.	____	____	____	____	____
5. My value as a person depends greatly on what others think of me.	____	____	____	____	____
6. I cannot find happiness without being loved by another person.	____	____	____	____	____
7. If others dislike you, you are bound to be less happy.	____	____	____	____	____
8. If people whom I care about reject me, it means there is something wrong with me.	____	____	____	____	____

Statement	Agree strongly	Agree slightly	Neutral	Disagree slightly	Disagree very much
9. If a person I love does not love me, it means I am unlovable.	_____	_____	_____	_____	_____
10. Being isolated from others is bound to lead to unhappiness.	_____	_____	_____	_____	_____
11. If I am to be a worthwhile person, I must be truly outstanding in at least one major respect.	_____	_____	_____	_____	_____
12. I must be a useful, productive, creative person or life has no purpose.	_____	_____	_____	_____	_____
13. People who have good ideas are more worthy than those who do not.	_____	_____	_____	_____	_____
14. If I do not do as well as other people, it means I am inferior.	_____	_____	_____	_____	_____
15. If I fail at my work, then I am a failure as a person.	_____	_____	_____	_____	_____
16. If you cannot do something well, there is little point in doing it at all.	_____	_____	_____	_____	_____
17. It is shameful for a person to display his or her weaknesses.	_____	_____	_____	_____	_____
18. A person should try to be the best at everything he or she undertakes.	_____	_____	_____	_____	_____
19. I should be upset if I make a mistake.	_____	_____	_____	_____	_____
20. If I don't set the highest standards for myself, I am likely to end up a second-rate person.	_____	_____	_____	_____	_____
21. If I strongly believe I deserve something, I have reason to expect I should get it.	_____	_____	_____	_____	_____
22. It is necessary to become frustrated if you find obstacles to getting what you want.	_____	_____	_____	_____	_____
23. If I put other people's needs before my own, they should help me when I need something from them.	_____	_____	_____	_____	_____

(cont.)

Statement	Agree strongly	Agree slightly	Neutral	Disagree slightly	Disagree very much
24. If I am a good husband or wife, then my spouse is bound to love me.	_____	_____	_____	_____	_____
25. If I do nice things for someone, I can anticipate that he or she will respect and treat me just as well as I treat them.	_____	_____	_____	_____	_____
26. I should assume responsibility for how people feel and behave if they are close to me.	_____	_____	_____	_____	_____
27. If I criticize the way someone does something and he or she becomes angry or depressed, this means I have upset him or her.	_____	_____	_____	_____	_____
28. To be a good, worthwhile, moral person, I must try to help everyone who needs it.	_____	_____	_____	_____	_____
29. If a child is having emotional or behavioral difficulties, this shows that the child's parents have failed in some important respect.	_____	_____	_____	_____	_____
30. I should be able to please everybody.	_____	_____	_____	_____	_____
31. I cannot expect to control how I feel when something bad happens.	_____	_____	_____	_____	_____
32. There is no point in trying to change upsetting emotions because they are a valid and inevitable part of daily living.	_____	_____	_____	_____	_____
33. My moods are primarily created by factors that are largely beyond my control, such as the past, body chemistry, hormone cycles, biorhythms, chance, or fate.	_____	_____	_____	_____	_____
34. My happiness is largely dependent on what happens to me.	_____	_____	_____	_____	_____
35. People who have the marks of success (good looks, social status, wealth, or fame) are bound to be happier than those who do not.	_____	_____	_____	_____	_____

Scoring the DAS

Now that you have completed the DAS, you can score it in the following way. Score your answer to each of the thirty-five attitudes according to this key:

Agree strongly	Agree slightly	Neutral	Disagree slightly	Disagree very much
−2	−1	0	+1	+2

Now add up your score on the first five attitudes. These measure your tendency to measure your worth in term of the opinions of others and the amount of approval or criticism you receive. Suppose your scores on these five items were +2, +1, −1, +2, 0. Then your total score for these five questions would be +4.

Proceed in this way to add up your score for items 1 through 5, 6 through 10, 11 through 15, 16 through 20, 21 through 25, 26 through 30, and 31 through 35, and record these as illustrated in the following example:

Scoring example:

Value system	Attitudes	Individual scores	Total score
I. Approval	1 through 5	+2, +1, −1, +2, 0	+4
II. Love	6 through 10	−2, −1, −2, −2, 0	−7
III. Achievement	11 through 15	+1, +1, 0, 0, −2	0
IV. Perfectionism	16 through 20	+2, +2, +1, +1, +1	+7
V. Entitlement	21 through 25	+1, +1, −1, +1, 0	+2
VI. Omnipotence	26 through 30	−2, −1, 0, −1, +1	−3
VII. Autonomy	31 through 35	−2, −2, −1, −2, −2	−9

Record your actual scores here:

Value system	Attitudes	Individual scores	Total score
I. Approval	1 through 5	_____	_____
II. Love	6 through 10	_____	_____
III. Achievement	11 through 15	_____	_____
IV. Perfectionism	16 through 20	_____	_____
V. Entitlement	21 through 25	_____	_____
VI. Omnipotence	26 through 30	_____	_____
VII. Autonomy	31 through 35	_____	_____

Each cluster of five items from the scale measures one of seven value systems. Your total score for each cluster of five items can range from +10 to −10. Now you can read about each variable and develop your personal philosophy profile.

Interpreting Your DAS Score

I. *Approval* (items 1–5): These items assess your tendency to base your self-esteem on others' reactions to you. A positive score (between 0 and +10) indicates that you are independent with a healthy sense of your own worth, even when confronted with criticism and disapproval. A negative score (between 0 and –10) indicates that you are very dependent, because you evaluate yourself through other people's eyes. You are vulnerable to anxiety and depression when others criticize you or are angry with you.

II. *Love* (items 6–10): These items assess your tendency to base your self-worth on whether or not you are loved. A positive score (between 0 and +10) indicates that you see love as desirable but that you have a wide range of other interests that you also find fulfilling and gratifying. Hence, love is not a requirement for your happiness or self-esteem. A negative score (between 0 and –10) indicates that you see love as a "need" without which you cannot survive or be happy. You tend to adopt inferior roles in relationships with people you care about for fear of alienating them. You may even resort to manipulative behavior in order to get people's affection and attention. Ironically, this needy, greedy attitude often drives people away, thus intensifying your loneliness.

III. *Achievement* (items 11–15): These items assess your tendency to base your self-esteem on whether or not you are productive. A positive score (between 0 and +10) indicates that you enjoy creativity and productivity but do not see them as a necessary road to self-esteem and satisfaction. A negative score (between 0 and –10) indicates that you are a workaholic. Your sense of self-worth and your capacity for joy are dependent on your productivity. If your business slumps, if you retire, or if you become ill or inactive, you will be at risk for an emotional crash.

IV. *Perfectionism* (items 16–20): These items assess your tendency to base your self-worth on your ability to avoid failures and mistakes. A positive score (between 0 and +10) indicates that you have the capacity to set meaningful, flexible, and appropriate standards. You enjoy processes and experiences for their own sake, and are not exclusively fixated on outcomes. You don't have to be outstanding at everything. You don't fear mistakes but see them as opportunities to grow and learn. A negative score (between 0 and –10) indicates that you demand perfection in yourself—mistakes are taboo, failure is "worse than death," and even negative emotions are a disaster. You are living with impossible and unrealistic personal standards, and life becomes a joyless, tedious treadmill.

V. *Entitlement* (items 21–25): These items measure the extent to which you feel you deserve the best out of life, simply because you're you. A positive score (between 0 and +10) indicates that you don't always feel automatically entitled to things, so you negotiate for what you want and often get it. You realize there is no inherent reason why things should always go your way. You experience a negative outcome as a disappointment, not a tragedy, knowing that you can't expect "justice" at all times. You are patient and persistent, with high frustration tolerance. A negative score (between 0 and –10) indicates that you feel entitled to things (success, love, happiness, etc.). You expect and demand that your wants be met by other people and the universe in general because of your inherent goodness and hard work. When this does not happen, you feel depressed and inadequate; you may become irate. Thus you expend much energy being frustrated, sad, and/or mad.

VI. *Omnipotence* (items 26–30): These items measure your tendency to see yourself as the center of your personal universe and to hold yourself responsible for much of what goes on around you. A positive score (between 0 and +10) indicates that you know the joy that comes from accepting that you are not the center of the universe. Since you are not in control of other adults, you are not ultimately responsible for them, but only for yourself. You relate to others as a collaborator. You aren't threatened when others disagree with your ideas or fail to follow your advice. People frequently listen to you and respect your ideas, because you do not polarize them with insistence that they must agree with you. Your relationships with people are characterized by mutuality instead of dependency. A negative score (between 0 and –10) indicates that you blame others who are not really under your control. Consequently, you are plagued by guilt and self-condemnation. The attitude that you should be omnipotent and all-powerful leaves you anxious and ineffective.

VII. *Autonomy* (items 31–35): These items measure your ability to find happiness within yourself. A positive score (between 0 and +10) indicates that all your moods are a result of your thoughts and attitudes. You assume responsibility for your feelings because you recognize that they are ultimately created by you. A negative score (between 0 and –10) indicates that you are trapped in the belief that your potential for joy and self-esteem comes from the outside. Your moods are the victim of external factors. This puts you at a disadvantage, because everything is ultimately beyond your control.

A Final Word on the DAS

The DAS is not an infallible test, and you may not agree with the results. If so, you're not alone; this questionnaire has been met with some of the strongest comments in our pain program. However, the overwhelming majority of people find the scale to be very valuable in identifying self-defeating attitudes, once their objections or their self-critical thoughts about the results ("I must really be crazy," "I didn't realize I was so dysfunctional") are put aside. It is amazing how accurately it identifies and predicts the types of scenarios that push people's vulnerable buttons. Give it a try.

Chapter 6

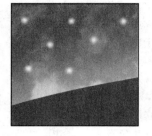

Adopting Healthy Attitudes

There was once an old farmer who had a mare. One day the mare broke through a fence and ran away. "Now you have no horse to pull your plow at planting time," the neighbors said. "What bad luck this is."

"Good luck, bad luck," replied the farmer. "Who knows?"

The next week the mare returned, bringing with her two wild stallions. "With three horses you are now a rich man," the neighbors said. "What good fortune this is."

"Good fortune, bad fortune," replied the farmer. "Who knows?"

That afternoon the farmer's only son tried to tame one of the stallions, but he was thrown and broke a leg. "Now you have no one to help you with planting," the neighbors said. "What bad luck this is."

"Good luck, bad luck," replied the farmer. "Who knows?"

The next day the emperor's soldiers rode into town and conscripted the oldest son of every family, but the farmer's son was left behind because of his broken leg. "Your son is the only eldest in the province who has not been taken from his family," the neighbors said. "What good fortune this is . . . "

—*A Zen story about an old Chinese farmer (retold in*
The Wellness Book, p. 460; see Chapter 2, "Supplementary Reading")

This Zen story characterizes a flexible attitude. In essence, it demonstrates that whatever people's interpretations of events may be, there is always considerable uncertainty in life. Developing an ease with uncertainty is a way of adapting to life's daily hassles and stresses. For people like you, who now find themselves living in pain, this adaptability can be crucial for coping. Medical and scientific research by Seligman (1998),

Fawzy et al. (1993), Nelson et al. (2000), and Williams and Williams (1998) has found that there are numerous health benefits for those who can shed rigid, destructive lifestyles, behaviors, and attitudes and adopt more flexible, positive ones. These benefits include decreased risk factors for heart disease, reduced recurrences of heart attacks, improved immune system function, and increased life span for cancer patients. Indeed, we are only just beginning to understand and appreciate the power of adaptability and positive attitudes.

The term "attitude" is used here to mean a psychological characteristic or posture that an individual usually adopts without thinking about it. Attitudes are the results of multiple factors, such as cultural influences, familial beliefs, learned behaviors, and perhaps genetics. We all have attitudes; they enable us to make our numerous daily decisions without consciously weighing every single one of them, and they influence our behaviors. Attitudes, however, can become problems when they are so negative and inflexible that they impair healthy functioning or prevent (or at least complicate) appropriate adaptation to the circumstances in which we find ourselves.

If, for example, you hold an attitude that you have no control over what happens to you, then you may find it difficult to see the benefit of engaging in healthy behaviors. You may say, "If I'm going to be in pain, why should I bother to stop smoking or follow a low-fat diet?" Or, to take another example, you may be in pain but may insist that you must continue housekeeping as you did before the pain. Chances are that you will suffer more and still not have a clean house. When you find yourself maintaining attitudes like these, you need to stop and examine them consciously.

The problematic attitudes of learned helplessness and of anger/hostility are common among the chronic pain patients I see. These particular attitudes are discussed here because they interfere to the greatest extent with effective coping and problem solving. By contrast, attitudes such as stress hardiness, optimism, empathy, and altruism can help ease the uncertainty of life in general and life with chronic pain in particular.

Problematic Attitudes

Learned Helplessness

If you put a rat in a cage and rig the cage so that every time the rat presses a bar it receives an electric shock, the rat will soon learn to avoid that behavior—pressing the bar. If a second rat's cage is connected to the first rat's cage so that every time Rat 1 presses the bar, Rat 2 gets a shock, Rat 2 will begin to act anxious and hypervigilant. Rat 2 has no control over what Rat 1 does, and therefore is not able to control the shocks it receives.

After a period of time in this uncertain and uncontrollable condition, if Rat 2 is put through a maze, it will not be able to learn new pathways as it did before. It will become withdrawn and may stop eating. If this goes on long enough, Rat 2 will make no effort to help itself even if the shocks have stopped. This behavior is called "learned helplessness." Because the rat has learned so thoroughly that there is nothing it can do to change its helpless circumstances, it allows that attitude to affect even the things over which it does have control.

Many patients experiencing chronic pain assume a similar attitude of learned helplessness. They may ask or even beg for help but find it difficult to believe that certain suggestions or techniques will alter the pain perception and help them gain control. This attitude, however, like the rat's, will only result in their getting more of the same ... nothing. Practicing the skills and performing the exploration tasks and other exercises in this book will allow you to identify areas in which you do have control and to learn new ways of living with pain.

Anger/Hostility

Anger and Responsibility

Chapter 5 mentions that working with feelings of anger requires a slightly different approach than just identifying or changing self-talk. Anger and hostility need to be explored in terms of a person's motivation for keeping them. Many times, anger and hostility involve blaming someone or something else as responsible for the feelings. The angry individual is trapped into holding onto the feelings because he or she does not feel responsible for them. This attitude, in turn, generates more of the same, as the solution *appears* to remain outside of the angry individual's control.

A person's need to hold someone or something responsible for his or her suffering can be very strong. Moreover, there are times when anger is both appropriate and justified. Anger is a very powerful emotion that can serve as a basis for constructive action and determination. But many studies, for example, of cardiovascular disease (see Williams and Williams in "Supplementary Reading"), have illustrated that simply holding onto anger or hostility, rather than using it as an impetus for constructive action, can be destructive to the victim. For one thing, as noted above, blaming others for one's misery only serves to give away the control you could have. For another, the held-onto anger spreads ever wider, causing depression, anxiety, self-doubt, and more anger.

Some people protest that accepting responsibility for the way they feel is equivalent to admitting that they have done something wrong or to giving in; this is definitely not the case, however. In addition, many angry patients have expressed a fear that if they let go of their anger there will be nothing left of them. The anger has become a self-sustaining force in their lives. Again, too, depression and anxiety often underlie the anger or are even created by it in many cases. Staying angry may help these patients to avoid facing such feelings. But who is it that is suffering by hanging on to such negative emotional states? As one patient said upon realizing the self-destructive nature of her anger, "I've been letting someone else live rent-free in my head!"

As noted in Chapter 5, patients whose pain is the result of injury from an accident at work or from someone else's negligence are understandably very angry at times. However, many patients involved in worker's compensation claims, litigation, or the like find themselves fighting against a mighty and invisible adversary. Their feelings of being wronged and misunderstood, and their attempts to find an explanation or compensation for the suffering, exacerbate the "me against them" attitude. For example, one of my patients was suing someone because she had slipped on the ice in that person's driveway and injured her back. I asked her whom she would have blamed if she had slipped on the ice in her own driveway. She replied without a pause, "Me, I guess."

Coping with anger involves identifying your own role or responsibilities in the process. One of these responsibilities may be to identify your automatic thoughts. For example, you may be thinking something like this: "Someone must pay for my suffering. The accident that injured me was an unforgivable event, and I will not be comforted until the wrong has been corrected." Once these thoughts have been divulged, it is necessary to identify where your responsibility ends and that of the others involved begins. Forgiveness may be characterized as the act of coming to acceptance of the injustices that you have incurred. It is a difficult and arduous process. However, it can help you clarify who's responsible for what after an injury.

The Five Phases of Forgiveness

Beverly Flanigan, a psychologist who has studied the process of forgiveness, describes five phases leading to forgiveness in her book *Forgiving the Unforgivable: Overcoming the Bitter Legacy of Intimate Wounds* (see "Supplementary Reading"). Although it is meant to be a description of forgiving betrayal and infidelity in personal relationships, the process she describes appears to be applicable to forgiving physical injuries as well.

Phase 1: Naming the Injury. The first phase gives you as the injured person the opportunity to clarify what the wrongful act was and to explore how you interpret the significance or meaning of that act.

For example, say the car you were driving was hit from behind and you received a neck injury. The wrongful act committed by the other driver was perhaps not leaving enough space between cars, speeding, or not paying attention to slowing traffic. When the significance of the wrongful act is explored, you may take it as a personal violation. Furthermore, if the other person has never apologized, you may feel further justified in seeking punishment for the person's wrongdoing. However, an implicit moral rule that may complicate your feelings about this act may be "Thou shalt do no harm."

If lawyers become involved, this important phase may be delayed until the case comes to court, many months or years later. As a result of not naming the injury and exploring its significance to you, you may also not be able to begin to admit that the painful consequences are permanent and take the steps necessary to cope with your new condition (Phase 2). In addition, the possibility of talking to the injurer will be limited to depositions, and you will be excluded from identifying or relating to any human weakness on his or her part (such as having made a mistake). Clearly, being wronged is painful; especially when the effects are physical and long term, there is a wish to be compensated at many levels. This is appropriate, but if the phases of forgiveness are arrested at the beginning, what may be experienced is that the external resolution (the settlement) is not accompanied by an internal resolution of the distress.

Phase 2: Claiming the Injury. If there is a progression to Phase 2, the process involves admitting that the injury is permanent and that the pain is yours to cope with. You stop blaming your suffering on the injurer, and you stop denying that you have the responsibility and need to go forward.

Phase 3: Blaming the Injurer. In Phase 3, someone is held accountable for causing the harm. In a situation involving a motor vehicle accident, such as the example given above, it is usually the other driver. Other situations involving injury may not be so clearcut. If you have experienced a work-related injury, it may be that the nature of the job—for example, the repetitive motion involved in typing at a word processor for long periods of time—has contributed to the injury. You may experience considerable frustration if you do not recover in the expected amount of time and can no longer perform your job. If you feel guilty or blamed for not returning to work, you may become angry at the workplace for not setting up the computer correctly in the first place.

In such cases, these feelings are often exacerbated by the lack of caring for a worker's physical and emotional needs. Although worker's compensation was originally designed as a sort of no-fault insurance for employers and their employees, this is rarely the case when chronic pain conditions occur. Once again, legal involvement may serve to delay resolution or to assign blame when actually none exists. Whereas assessing blame may be appropriate in cases of harm resulting from negligence, accidents, or assault, it may not always be possible in cases of chronic pain. If you are a pain patient in such circumstances, it is important to avoid assigning blame inappropriately (to either yourself or others) and to realize that you can move on to the next phase as well.

Phase 4: Balancing the Scales. When the need to take responsibility for coping with the injury has been admitted (Phase 2), and the question of who, if anyone, needs to be held responsible for causing the injury has been resolved (Phase 3), then forgiving can proceed. Forgiving begins from a position of strength. If you continue to feel powerless to cope with your pain, then the anger you feel may perpetuate the helplessness and hopelessness of being a victim. Identifying with the responsibility to *live with* the pain, as opposed to responsibility for *causing* the pain, can enable you to cope from a position of self-awareness. If you are aware of your feelings and motivations, you can identify where your responsibilities end and those of others begin, thus balancing the scale.

When an injurer is found to be responsible, then punishment through the courts and restitution, not revenge or recrimination, is in order. This was probably the original role of the legal system in such circumstances.

Phase 5: Choosing to Forgive. The art of forgiving implies that you are ready to let go of the negative feelings that until now have imprisoned your mind, spirit, and heart. In so doing, you move toward repairing the injury by moving on with the life you have now. Forgiveness is coming to acceptance of your new life, even if it is one of pain. Through this process, forgivers find and create new answers that, in a way, make them new people. "If nothing can ever be the same, this time around, perhaps it can be better" (Flanigan, 1992, p. 162).

Writing the Wrongs

The writing exercise mentioned in the "Exploration Tasks" of Chapter 5 has been helpful to people who have trouble identifying the thoughts behind their anger and the motivational factors behind their thoughts. Begin by asking yourself, "Who has hurt me and what have they done?" Then list what you gain by staying angry and what you gain by giving it up. Compare the two sides of your list. What are your conclusions?

Healthy Attitudes

Much of behavioral research to date has focused primarily on describing negative attitudes and their relationship to ill health. However, explorations by some researchers have identified various attitudes that are associated with positive health outcomes.

Stress Hardiness

Suzanne Kobasa of the University of Chicago, for example, studied "stress-hardy" executives—ones who exhibited an attitude of challenge, commitment, and control—and found that they experienced fewer physical and emotional symptoms during a particularly stressful business period than those who didn't. She found that the stress-hardy executives viewed life changes as challenges rather than as threats; they felt committed to their work, as well as to their families and social institutions. They also believed that their response to whatever happened was within their control.

Another researcher who has examined positive health attitudes is Aaron Antonovsky of the Ben-Gurion University of the Negev in Israel. Antonovsky talked with a group of Holocaust survivors in Israel who appeared to have remained in good emotional health in spite of their having experienced terrible trauma. From his discussions with these exceptional survivors and others, Antonovsky has gone on to develop his theory of the "sense of coherence." He has proposed that people with a high sense of coherence have a pervasive, enduring, yet dynamic feeling of confidence that (1) stressors coming from the internal and external environments are structured, predictable, and explicable; (2) they themselves have resources available to meet the demands resulting from these stressors; and (3) these demands are challenges worthy of investment and engagement.

Optimism

Optimism, too, has been declared a healthy attitude. Optimists are those individuals who anticipate the best outcome and expect pleasurable experiences to occur. Optimism has been associated with an enhanced immune system, and Sandra Levy, a psychoneuroimmunologist, has shown an optimistic explanatory style to be a strong predictor of the length of cancer remission (see Hafen et al. in "Supplementary Reading"). Martin Seligman has demonstrated that a pessimistic style is associated with depression and general poor health. Pessimists see events that happen to them as stable ("This *always* happens to me"), global ("I *never* do anything right"), and internal ("It's all *my* fault"). In contrast, optimists see events as unstable ("Just because it happened once doesn't mean it will again"), specific ("I have trouble with pacing my activities"), and external ("Other people are responsible for their behaviors, I'm responsible for mine").

Empathy

There are several definitions of the word "empathy." Here, it is used to mean a *nonjudgmental* awareness of others' experience. Remember the excerpt from Joan's writing exercise at the beginning of Chapter 5? If you were able to come to some understanding of what Joan was experiencing, you were feeling empathy. If, on the other hand, you found yourself making derogatory or unflattering comments, then you were judging.

If we are asked to judge, to assess the content of our thoughts, then judgment is in order. But many times we are too quick to judge. This leaves us vulnerable to rash decisions, such as assuming that a situation or individual has no redeeming qualities; it also decreases our options to explore further explanations or possibilities. We can have a strong tendency to make judgments quickly, particularly if we are feeling out of control.

Suspending judgment may at first seem too open-ended; it may apparently require you to remain in an eternal state of ambiguity. Actually, it gives you the time necessary to gather information, to walk in the other person's shoes, and to experience various viewpoints. It also allows a certain level of patience for others, and ultimately for yourself. When you begin to realize that as humans we suffer a lot from basing our judgments on illusions and misinformation and that we only *think* we know what's going on, you can begin to relax about the long process necessary for change. Being more relaxed about this process allows you to suspend the tendency to evaluate your efforts as good or bad, right or wrong, and to explore the wide range of possibilities and choices that lie before you.

As noted at the beginning of this chapter, such flexibility is a key component of the positive attitudes that have been identified to enhance our health and lives.

Altruism

A rabbi had a conversation with the Lord about Heaven and Hell. "I will show you Hell," said the Lord, and led the rabbi into a room in the middle of which was a very big round table. The people sitting at it were starving and desperate.

In the middle of the room was an enormous pot of stew, more than enough for everyone. The smell of the stew was delicious and made the rabbi's mouth water. The people around the table were holding spoons with very long handles. Each person found that it was just possible to reach the pot to take a spoonful of the stew, but because the handle of the spoon was longer than anyone's arm, no one could get the food into his mouth.

The rabbi saw that their suffering was indeed terrible. "Now I will show you Heaven," said the Lord, and they went into another room which was exactly the same as the first room.

There was the same big round table and the same enormous pot of stew. The people, as before, were equipped with the same long-handled spoons. But here they were well nourished and plump, laughing, and talking.

At first the rabbi could not understand. "It is simple, but requires a certain skill," said the Lord. "You see, they have learned to feed each other." (Jewish folk tale)*

As human beings, we need each other. Nurturing this connectedness can be very difficult when you are in pain, because pain can preoccupy you to such an extent that it shuts your eyes to the needs of others. Once you have established what kind of pacing of activities you require, think seriously about joining a support group, volunteering, or getting involved with a political passion you may have, so as to help fulfill someone else's needs.

Building a Foundation for Attitude Change

> Assume a virtue, though you have it not. . . . Refrain tonight;
> And that shall lend a kind of easiness to the next abstinence: the
> next more easy;
> For practice can almost change the stamp of nature.
> —*William Shakespeare,* Hamlet

If you don't already have them, it is possible to develop healthier attitudes such as stress hardiness, optimism, empathy, and altruism. Attitudes are not fixed or unchangeable. It is possible to alter the filters through which you see your world. The skills presented throughout this book can help you explore and develop the qualities of positive, healthy attitudes.

The following techniques in particular will help you work on developing healthier attitudes. Affirmations can encourage your positive self-talk and nurture your self-esteem; examining the sources of your self-esteem can help strengthen your courage and fortitude; and humor can ease the hard work of change.

Affirmations

Chapter 5 discusses ways of changing negative self-talk; up to this point, this chapter has discussed how certain positive or negative attitudes affect the way you feel about the world around you. You can use "affirmations" to change your attitudes in a positive way. Affirmations are generally short positive statements, quotes, or reflections that you can repeat to yourself and that make you feel inspired, comforted, or supported.

There are many ways of using and developing affirmations. You may want to refer to a book that provides daily reflections (e.g., see Schaef in "Supplementary Reading") or to spiritual books for inspiration. Or you may select a quote, phrase, or passage that simply

*Retold by Irvin D. Yalom in *The Theory and Practice of Group Psychotherapy,* Third Edition (New York: Basic Books, 1975, pp. 12–13).

comes to mind during the day's activities. Perhaps you may find that an affirmation comes to you at the end of an RR technique (see Chapter 3). You may not always agree at first with this spontaneous affirmation, but if you repeat it throughout the day, you may find that it inspires you to consider a feeling or attitude you wish to develop.

For example, you may end your RR technique with the statement "I am strong." It arises from your unconscious, but your more conscious self says, "Who are you kidding? I don't feel strong at all! I'm the original 120-pound weakling!" As you contemplate or repeat the affirmation "I am strong" periodically for a week, however, you may begin to appreciate that you are getting in touch with qualities of strength that are not physical in nature; that is, you are developing strength of courage, fortitude, and will. You feel inspired to do more with your life as a result. Many times, as in this case, the most useful and relevant affirmations are those you generate yourself.

Write out a few affirmations that come to you during the next week while you are practicing an RR technique. Post them on the refrigerator or on the dashboard of your car so that you can be reminded of them. See what happens.

Examining the Sources of Self-Esteem

Self-esteem, or the way you feel about yourself, is the end result of many factors. The DAS (see Chapter 5) can help you to identify the unchallenged assumptions you may hold that make adapting to life stressors more difficult. The following exercise can also help you determine and strengthen your vulnerable areas.

Write out 10 things that you like about yourself:

1. _____
2. _____
3. _____
4. _____
5. _____
6. _____
7. _____
8. _____
9. _____
10. _____

Now, write out 10 things that you don't like about yourself or feel you would like to change:

1. _____
2. _____

3. _____

4. _____

5. _____

6. _____

7. _____

8. _____

9. _____

10. _____

Which list was easier to complete? Why?

_____

_____

If you're like most people, the negative things are easier to get in touch with. Saying what you like about yourself is often labeled as conceited or self-centered, so you may feel compelled to qualify positive statements with "but" or "not always." Remember, however: It's okay to feel satisfied with something you do, feel, or like about yourself.

Look at the list that contains things you like about yourself. Put a check (√) next to those things that are internal characteristics ("patience," "compassionate," "good listener"). Put an (×) next to those characteristics that are external ("good worker," "good friend," "pretty face"). Is there a balance of (√) and (×), or are you heavy on the (×) side?

Traits that are external are more vulnerable to the judgments of others and to losses (e.g., loss of job, good health, or personal relations). Many people in pain suffer even more when their major source of self-esteem resides in what they do (or did) for a career or for the outside world. It's important for individuals to have both internal and external qualities on which to build their self-esteem. It creates a firm foundation for becoming engaged with the world around them.

See whether you can balance your list of positive traits with both external and internal attributes. Are there any traits on your negative list that you might turn into positive traits through goal setting?

Humor

Just as self-esteem diminishes in many of those who experience chronic pain, so does the ability to see the humor in themselves and the world around them. The preoccupation with self and the sadness associated with grieving for the loss of "normal" functioning can make it difficult to find the humor in life. To be able to use humor implies a healthy mind–body interaction; this does not mean that you have to be pain free.

In Chapter 5, you may have found yourself chuckling while identifying your automatic thoughts. You may have wondered, "Now where in the world did I get *that* idea?!"

Laughing at your own follies and foibles is healthy and can generate positive attitudes that last long after the laugh. It helps to insure flexibility and reminds you not to take everything so seriously. In fact, laughter is thought to enhance the production of endorphins (the body's natural opiates), which can diminish pain awareness.

Like any behavior, the use of humor, especially wisecracking, can be used to hide underlying negative attitudes that need to be explored. Good-natured conscious giggling, on the other hand, is not only desirable, it is necessary. It's also important to be able to laugh spontaneously. Indeed, real life's challenges to our assumptions and expectations are often the source of our biggest laughs.

If you are finding it hard to find something to laugh about, watch a funny movie; read a favorite book of cartoons; read the writings of Loretta Laroche or other astute life observers; buy a joke book; or, if you really get stuck, watch small children at play. Somehow, adulthood becomes "a-dolt-hood" for too many of us. Commit yourself now to consciously seeking out a giggle, if not an outright guffaw, on at least a weekly basis.

Summary

- Making changes in negative lifestyles, behaviors, and attitudes has been found to result in a number of specific health benefits and can greatly improve your ability to cope with chronic pain.
- An attitude is a psychological characteristic or posture that can result from various factors but that is generally adopted unconsciously by an individual.
- Holding on to certain negative attitudes can impair healthy functioning and prevent appropriate adaptation to new circumstances. Such attitudes need to be examined consciously.
- Learned helplessness can paralyze you to such an extent that you cannot work on healing. Remember that you do have choices and you do have control.
- Anger has a place, but holding on to it is destructive. Forgiveness is one way of coping effectively with anger; there are five phases for forgiveness.
- Studies of stress-hardy and optimistic individuals indicate that these attitudes are associated with healthier coping and functioning.
- Empathy is a nonjudgmental understanding of what someone is feeling; it can help you avoid rash decisions and can increase your options.
- Altruism is an important way of staying connected with others.
- Affirmations are short, positive statements, quotes, or reflections that you can repeat to yourself for inspiration, comfort, or support.
- Self-esteem is how you feel about yourself. Most people find it easier to get in touch with their negative characteristics than with their positive ones; however, emphasizing your positive traits will enhance your self-esteem.
- Conscious humor is healthy. It is associated with the production of endorphins and generates positive attitudes that last long after the laugh.

Exploration Tasks

1. Continue recording your automatic thoughts associated with negative emotional states (see Chapter 5). Identify the distortions and their possible sources through your own explorations. Change the automatic thoughts to reflect the reality of the situation, using any of the three reframing techniques discussed in Chapter 5. Copy and use the worksheet at the back of the book to record your explorations in negative self-talk. As you employ the techniques suggested in the present chapter, do you find your self-talk becoming more positive?

2. Continue with your practice of the basic RR techniques (1–5) on a daily basis. As suggested in the text, use phrases and statements that come to you during your RR practice as personal affirmations.

3. Write out a goal that you want to accomplish related to the material in this chapter. As always, make sure your goal is a behavioral task that you can measure in terms of the steps *you* will take to accomplish it. Here is an example:

Goal: *To do something that makes me laugh at least once a week.*

Steps to take to reach that goal:

A. *Read The New Yorker.*

B. *Rent a humorous video.*

C. *Read the newspaper cartoons.*

Now it's your turn.

Goal: _____

Steps to take to reach that goal:

A. _____

B. _____

C. _____

D. _____

In addition, list contingency plans. That is, identify what obstacles might get in the way of your accomplishing this goal. What solutions can you devise to work toward insuring the success of this goal?

Obstacles	**Solutions**
A. _____	_____
B. _____	_____
C. _____	_____
D. _____	_____

Supplementary Reading

The following books provide additional information on attitudes and how to change them:

Fawzy I. Fawzy, Nancy Fawzy, Christine Hyun, Robert Elashoff, Donald Guthrie, John Fahey, and Donald Morton, "Malignant Melanoma: Effects of an Early Structured Psychiatric Intervention, Coping, and Affective State on Recurrence and Survival 6 Years Later," *Archives of General Psychiatry, 50*: 681–688, 1993.

Beverly Flanigan, *Forgiving the Unforgivable: Overcoming the Bitter Legacy of Intimate Wounds* (New York: Macmillan, 1992).

Brent Q. Hafen, Kathryn J. Frandsen, Keith J. Karren, and Keith Hooker, *The Health Effects of Attitudes, Emotions and Relationships* (Provo, UT: EMS, 1992).

Allen Klein, *The Healing Power of Humor* (Los Angeles: Tarcher, 1989).

Suzanne Kobasa, "Stressful Life Events, Personality and Health: An Inquiry into Hardiness," *Journal of Personality and Social Psychology, 37:* 1–11, 1979.

Loretta Laroche, *Life Is Not a Stress Rehearsal: Bringing Yesterday's Sane Wisdom into Today's Insane World* (New York: Broadway Books, 2001).

Miriam Nelson, Wendy Wray, and Sarah Wernick, *Strong Women Stay Young* (New York: Bantam Doubleday Dell Publications, 2000).

Robert Ornstein and David Sobel, *Healthy Pleasures* (Reading, MA: Perseus Books, 1990).

Anne Wilson Schaef, *Meditations for Women Who Do Too Much* (San Francisco: Harper, 1996).

Martin Seligman, *Learned Optimism* (New York: Pocket Books, 1998).

Idries Shah, *The Pleasantries of the Incredible Mulla Nasrudin* (London: Octagon Press, 1983).

Idries Shah, *Reflections* (London: Octagon Press, 1983).

Idries Shah, *The Subtleties of the Inimitable Mulla Nasrudin* and *The Exploits of the Incomparable Mulla Nasrudin* (London: Octagon Press, 1989).

Redford B. Williams and Virginia Williams, *Anger Kills: Seventeen Strategies for Controlling the Hostility That Can Harm Your Health* (New York: Harper Mass Market Paperback, 1998).

Denise Winn, *The Manipulated Mind: Brainwashing, Conditioning and Manipulation*(Los Altos, CA: Malor Books, 2000).

Chapter 7

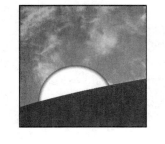

Nutrition and Pain

Why Discuss Nutrition?

Why include a chapter on nutrition in a pain management book? Well, there are three reasons. First, good nutritional habits, like exercise and relaxation techniques, are essential for good health; the program described in this book treats the whole person, as well as the pain. Second, some specific nutritional behaviors can affect pain levels (these are discussed in more detail later). Third, there is a great deal of misinformation at present about nutritional therapies for pain. This last point deserves additional comment here.

The United States as a culture is obsessed with diets, body weight, and food; few Americans consider eating simply as the partaking of basic sustenance. Because food is so accessible, and eating habits are such a national obsession, food remedies, diets, and supplements are eagerly adopted by the public. In addition, there has been a growing dissatisfaction with organized medicine, particularly in treating chronic disease. Patients are increasingly willing to embrace such "natural," "holistic" therapies as megadose vitamin therapy, fasting, and internal cleansing. The language used to justify the claims for some of these nutritional treatments sounds scientific, but there is rarely evidence other than patients' personal testimonials to support their claims.

Here are just some of the difficulties encountered in studies of nutritional therapies, which are the reasons that such studies must be designed and evaluated carefully. An examination of research papers on the process of digestion and absorption of food components makes it apparent that the whole process of nutrition is not a simple one. For example, some food components are only absorbed when needed by the body, and others are absorbed only if there are other essential components available in the same meal. Add to that the complexity of asking every single participant in a nutritional study to eat the same thing, while meeting individual metabolic needs, for a long enough time to see changes in symptoms, and you can see that the task is formidable.

The most common pain syndrome that has received consideration regarding dietary influences is rheumatoid arthritis. The research has involved three lines of investigation: fish and plant oils, vegetarian/fasting diets, and hypersensitivity/food allergies. The strongest evidence supports the intake of fish oils that contain omega-3 polyunsaturated fatty acids. Studies show that concentrated fish oil supplements, about 3 grams a day, were associated with decreased inflammation and pain in patients with rheumatoid arthritis. Fish oil has not been shown to benefit osteoarthritis. Plant oils that are considered to promote anti-inflammatory effects are flaxseed (1 to 3 tablespoons per day), a source of eicosapentaenoic acid (EPA), and evening primrose oil and borage oil, a source of gamma-linoleic acid (GLA), at 1.8 grams per day. The amounts needed for effectiveness of these specific fatty acids are also associated with blood thinning, so check with your doctor if you are planning to take these supplements and are on anti-inflammatory drugs or blood-thinning drugs (e.g., Coumadin®), or using ginger or tumeric.

The other investigations have produced mixed results regarding their effects on symptoms of rheumatoid arthritis. The most that can and should be said at this time about special diets is that some people with rheumatoid arthritis appear to benefit from eliminating dairy products, reducing saturated fats, which are higher in nonvegetarian diets, and eliminating certain foods such as wheat, corn, peanuts, or eggs or some food additives or seasonings (MSG [monosodium glutamate]). Elimination diets to test food sensitivities are complicated to institute and should be undertaken with the supervision of a dietitian and/or doctor who is experienced in such diets. See "Supplementary Reading" for more detailed references on these topics.

In the other chronic pain syndromes, there is almost no firm evidence that food allergies play a role or that improvements can be obtained with extreme dietary supplementation (e.g., megadoses of vitamins or minerals or extracts of animal hormones and herbs) or elimination (e.g., yeast-free diets). In other words, research has simply not obtained sufficient proof that such treatments work to warrant recommending them to patients. Indeed, there is often potential harm (including dietary deficiencies, imbalances, and toxicities, as well as enormous financial costs to patients) associated with such treatments. I do endorse the careful study of nutritional therapies, and I recommend keeping an open mind to the possibility that in the future some patients will be able to control their pain symptoms with dietary manipulation.

In the interim, while we're all awaiting further clarification, you can begin following some basic nutritional recommendations now to improve your general health and help you in your pain management. These are explored in the following pages.

Two Important Principles

The basic approach to nutrition taken here can be summarized in the following two slogans: "Fresh is best" and "Moderation." These two simple recommendations may be more difficult to follow than you think—especially given the ease and wide availability of prepared foods and fast foods in the United States; the frantic pace of Americans' busy lives, which leaves little time for meal preparations; and the soothing feeling that many people in pain get from eating.

"Fresh is best" is a reminder that the more our foods are prepared by others before they reach our households, the more likely they are to have added salt, sugar, saturated fats, preservatives, and artificial coloring. In addition, increased processing may decrease fiber and nutritional content. Much of this manipulation of food is the result of processing foods to give them a longer shelf life, as well as to meet the appetite of the average American consumer, who has been eating a diet high in fat and sodium and low in fiber for quite a while. However, there is increasing evidence that low-fiber, high-fat, and high-sodium diets may put individuals at risk for developing heart disease, some cancers (colon cancer), high blood pressure, and obesity. Obesity can increase the risk of degenerative joint disease, osteoarthritis, particularly in the lower extremities; this is of particular concern to people already experiencing chronic pain, as it can complicate the pain management problem further.

"Moderation" is a fairly open-ended term that probably can best be interpreted by the end result—a stable weight that is appropriate for your height and body type. Eating at regular times, from a variety of foods in the four basic food groups (discussed below), and in quantities that meet the caloric requirements of your activities and metabolism will help you maintain a stable weight. Realizing that habits like skipping meals, eating your largest meal in the evening, or snacking on high-fat foods (chips, ice cream, cakes, or candy) contribute to weight problems will also help you maintain moderation in your diet. The body appears to have a natural wisdom that enables it to pick and choose what it needs, when it needs it, if it is not overwhelmed by excess.

Basic Nutritional Guidelines

The American diet continues to be associated with increasing obesity, heart disease, and stroke. Over the past decade, the U.S. Department of Agriculture, U.S. Department of Health and Human Services, and the American Heart Association have made recommendations for altering what we eat. The most recent recommendations have simplified the information to encourage adoption of a diet that would serve to decrease weight, saturated fats, cholesterol, and portion amounts.

1. *Portion amounts.* Picture a dinner plate that is divided in half. One half of the plate represents the amount of fruits and vegetables you should eat. One quarter of the remaining plate is the portion of meat or meat substitute (the size of a deck of cards), and the other quarter is the whole grains/starch portion.

2. *Healthy eating.* Eat a variety of fruits, vegetables, whole grains, legumes (beans), fish, lean meat, and poultry. Each day eat five servings of vegetables and fruits and six servings of grain products (including whole grains). Eat two servings of a fatty fish per week. Use fat-free and low-fat dairy products.

3. *Weight loss (and maintaining a normal weight).* Weight loss helps protect the weight-bearing joints from deterioration, but it is also important for a healthy lifestyle. To lose weight you must eat *fewer* calories than you burn. So, you can increase activities that increase calorie demands—aerobic exercise and strengthening (resistance training) exercises—or decrease your calorie intake.

Additional recommendations for healthy eating and weight loss include reducing or eliminating sweet soft drinks and commercially prepared baked goods; increasing exercise to 30 minutes a day of brisk walking or comparable activity or at least 180 minutes per week of combined activity/exercise. Resistance training has been shown to be a most beneficial way of increasing metabolism. This can be accomplished by doing up to three sets of 12 repetitions each with five to six muscle groups using three- to five-pound weights every other day.

Plan on a gradual weight loss of one to two pounds per week. Although this may seem slow, it will result in a more sustained weight loss. Because prevention of obesity is easier than losing weight, the recommendations for healthy diet, activity, and portion size will all be helpful if followed before a weight problem occurs.

Basic Food Group Nutrients

The four basic food groups are:

- Fruits and vegetables
- Whole grain products, cereals, and breads
- Low-fat dairy products
- Lean meat, poultry, fish and other meat substitutes (e.g., beans or legumes, soybean curd, or tofu, and eggs)

They provide us with the following nutrients:

- Carbohydrates
- Proteins
- Fats
- Vitamins and minerals

Carbohydrates

Carbohydrates are classified as either "simple" or "complex." Simple carbohydrates are sugars, such as table sugar, honey, and syrups. It is recommended that simple sugars be used in moderation—that is, in small amounts. Though sugar has a bad reputation in U.S.

culture, the main problem for adults is the company it keeps, such as the fat in pastries and ice cream. Eating fresh fruit can satisfy a sweet tooth and is a healthier choice.

Complex carbohydrates are made up of repeating chains of sugar molecules. Starch is an example of a complex carbohydrate. Vegetables and grains are excellent sources of complex carbohydrates, as well as of fiber, vitamins, and iron.

Proteins

Proteins are made up of amino acid units. The amino acid units are used by the body after being broken down in digestion; they are either metabolized for energy or reassembled into new proteins. Proteins are the building blocks of enzymes, hormones, and muscle tissue. The meat/meat substitutes group is a good source of proteins. Note that meat substitutes include legumes (dried beans and peas), tofu (soybean curd), fish, shellfish, eggs, and nuts. Meat as a food source is inherently good, but it has fallen into disrepute because it can contain a lot of hormones and antibiotics (given to animals while alive), it is a source of saturated fat and cholesterol, and in the past it was associated with diets of little nutritional variety ("meat and potatoes"). In addition, for a variety of reasons (including religious convictions, the rising financial and ecological costs of meat, and growing sensitivity to animal rights), increasing numbers of people are choosing to make use of meat substitutes.

Fats

Fats are made up of substances called "fatty acids" and "glycerol. " Fatty acids can be saturated, polyunsaturated, or monounsaturated; the less they are saturated, the healthier they are. Glycerol is the "carrier" that binds fatty acids together. Fats are used for energy and are easily stored in the body, and we all know their favorite storage places—the thighs, abdomen, and buttocks.

As mentioned earlier, there are fatty acids associated with production of inflammatory products. These omega-6 linoleic fatty acids are commonly found in corn and safflower oil, and they are converted to arachidonic acids that are converted to "bad" leukotrienes and prostaglandins that cause inflammation. The omega-3 linoleic fatty acids found in fish oils, flaxseed, and soybeans contain EPA and DHA that help form the "good" prostaglandins and leukotrienes that reduce inflammation. If your chronic pain has a component of inflammation, you may find that changing the balance to omega-3 fatty acids from omega-6 fatty acids to be helpful. Even if your pain is not due to inflammation, there is evidence that such dietary changes in the type of fatty acids you consume can help your heart health and may help prevent some cancers (colon).

The best source of fish oils is cold-water fish (sardines, trout, salmon). Capsules of fish oil, borage, and evening primrose oil (that contain gamma-linoleic acid) are available to supplement the diet, but large numbers of capsules a day are required to alter the fatty acid balance, and the expense may be prohibitive. As with many dietary recommendations, it may be better to alter what you eat to include the recommendations already made for healthy eating than to depend on supplements in an unhealthy diet.

Cholesterol is not a fat; it is a substance present in some foods, such as eggs, dairy products, and animal fats (always animal products). The intake of fat and cholesterol in the diet contributes to the body's production of cholesterol. This is the reason you hear the terms "cholesterol" and "fats" together so often. There are several types of cholesterol, and too much cholesterol of one type (low-density lipoprotein, or LDL) can contribute to diseases such as atherosclerosis (hardening of the arteries) or gallstones.

Vitamins and Minerals

Vitamins and minerals are food elements that are necessary in very small amounts for the normal functioning of many body processes. They are essential in the diet because the body is either unable to make them or makes them in insufficient amounts. Vegetables and grains are good sources of vitamins. There is considerable controversy regarding the benefit of supplemental vitamins and minerals in health and disease. For a normal healthy adult, eating a variety of foods should provide the essential nutrients from which the body can choose what is needed when it is needed. No research has disputed this to date. What are the needs of a stressed or ill body? These remain to be defined, and much more extensive exploration of the topic is needed.

Managing Pain through Nutrition

> What is food to one, is to others bitter poison.
> —*Lucretius (circa 94–55 B.C.)*

Although the principles and requirements presented above should serve to direct your basic nutritional choices, there is room for a great deal of individual variation. Everyone has different digestive and metabolic rates, genetic compositions, and activity levels, all of which affect food requirements. The various conflicting and sometimes dangerous diet trends or fads should be approached with caution. The top two pain syndromes that have received the most attention in terms of food-related symptom worsening are rheumatoid arthritis, discussed earlier, and migraine headaches.

Again, there does appear to be an internal body wisdom. If you do not ignore these signals, such as increasing pain, fatigue, or indigestion after eating or drinking certain foods or beverages, you can learn from your body. Just as you should learn to listen to your pain and distress, you should heed your body's signals associated with eating. This will help you to understand how you eat, when you eat, what you eat, and why you eat.

Because certain foods and beverages are associated with increasing pain in some individuals, keeping a food diary similar to your pain diary (one is provided at the back of the book) can be a useful way to identify patterns. For example, have you found yourself avoiding certain drinks or foods because of your pain? If so, what do you avoid? Or do you find yourself eating more of a certain food group? If so, what foods are these?

Behavioral "Appetizers" and "Desserts"

We Americans live in a fast-paced, high-stress society, and for those who have the added challenge of being in pain, it is particularly important to take the proper time to prepare to eat.

Before you begin your meal, take a few moments to smell the aromas and look at the colors of the food before you. Saying grace or giving thanks may be a way to allow you to pause in this manner before taking your nourishment.

Try, when possible, to eat without distractions. Avoid eating with a newspaper, a magazine, or the television in front of you. Notice what it feels like just to eat. Are you bored or anxious? Or does it feel pleasurable?

After eating, take a few moments to read, share a pleasurable activity, or daydream as your body digests its food. If you feel uncomfortable or bloated, or have indigestion, it may reflect what you've eaten or how you've eaten. These are important cues to document in your diary.

When to Eat

Many of us eat on a relatively uneven or arbitrary schedule. Some people eat between meals because those are the times they find themselves hungry or bored. Others skip meals and consume most of their calories in the evening.

It has long been known that breaking your night's fasting by eating a good breakfast (literally, "break-fast") is a healthy thing to do, because it supplies your body with the energy to start your daily activities. Skipping breakfast tends to result in bad nutritional habits, such as grabbing doughnuts, candy, or soft drinks later in the morning. If individuals who are prone to hypoglycemia (low blood sugar) do this, they will experience mood swings, irritability, and increased pain, which will then be relieved again by sweets—only to recur with even greater intensity several hours later.

Hypoglycemia is a condition that may be experienced by those with a family history of diabetes, but this is not always the case. Many physicians deny that the condition exists or has any discernable symptoms, though its presence is documentable by glucose tolerance tests. It is exacerbated by prolonged fasting periods. Susceptible individuals find that when they eat sweets in isolation as described above, they experience symptoms an hour or two later that are thought to be due to low blood sugar. In addition to the mood symptoms noted above, shakiness, sweating, headaches, muscle aches, and fatigue may result. Snack on fruit or yogurt instead of candy bars and eat small, frequent meals, thus avoiding prolonged periods of fasting. Several patients with headaches and fibromyalgia found that their symptoms improved after they followed these recommendations.

Eating the largest meal of the day in the evening is also not conducive to using the nutrients for energy. It may contribute to weight gain, poor sleep, and reflux (the movement of acid from the stomach back into the esophagus) if sleep follows too closely after the evening meal.

What to Eat and Why

Once again, eating a variety of fresh foods in moderation is the key to healthy eating. If you need to lose weight, watch the fat content of your foods, exercise, and consume moderate portions. Identifying what you eat and noting any corresponding increase or decrease in your pain can also help you determine which foods, ingredients, or additives to avoid and which foods to keep in your diet. (Some specific suggestions are provided below.)

Identifying why you eat is also critical, because many people who have pain report that eating makes them feel good, at least temporarily. Eating is thought to release endorphins (the body's own painkillers), which may explain this good feeling. So considering how eating makes you feel may give you important clues to get the most out of your diet. You may find, for instance, that you overeat for comfort. Nurturing yourself in other ways—through practicing RR techniques, becoming aware of other pleasurable activities, and seeking social support—may help reduce your need for "comfort eating."

Food Ingredients/Additives Linked to Increases in Pain

Let's take a look at the following culprits that have been associated with increases in pain sensation:

- Caffeine
- Alcohol
- Monosodium glutamate (MSG)
- Aspartame

Caffeine. Caffeine is an addictive stimulant, so it is advisable to consider decreasing your caffeine intake when you are under a lot of stress or in pain. But be careful: You can experience headaches and fatigue if you suddenly stop drinking caffeinated beverages altogether. Instead of stopping abruptly, you should gradually decrease your intake to avoid withdrawal symptoms. For example, instead of having five cups of coffee each morning, try two cups of decaffeinated coffee and three cups of regular coffee for a week. Next, continue to decrease the number of cups of regular coffee until you are drinking only decaffeinated coffee. Then decrease the number of cups of decaf as well, if you wish.

Caffeine is naturally present in coffee, tea, chocolate, and cocoa. It is also found in some soft drinks (such as colas) and in many prescription and nonprescription drugs (particularly cold, pain, stimulant, and weight-control preparations). The following table shows how caffeine levels can vary, depending on the type of beverage and how it is prepared.

Caffeine Content of Common Beverages

Beverage	Measure	Caffeine (mg)
Coffee		
Brewed, ground	8 ounces	80–200*
Instant	1 teaspoon	50–66
Decaffeinated	1 teaspoon	2–5
Tea (regular bag)		20–100*
Brewed 3 minutes		36
Brewed 5 minutes		46
Soft drinks		
Colas	12 ounces	43–65
Hot cocoa	8 ounces	5–10

*The longer the coffee and tea are brewed, the greater the caffeine content.

Alcohol. Alcohol is a blood vessel dilator and therefore may trigger migraines or exacerbate existing headaches. An earlier theory, which explained that migraines were caused by blood vessel dilatation following intense blood vessel constriction, is now known to be inaccurate or at best inadequate. However, some migraine sufferers may find that alcohol is best left alone, whatever the underlying mechanism may be. Other substances that may dilate blood vessels are tyramine and histamine. Tyramine can be found in red wine and some cheeses; histamine can be found in some wines and champagnes. (See the article by Radnitz in "Supplementary Reading.")

Many other patients in pain also find an association between pain and alcohol use. If you do *not* find that your pain improves when alcohol is eliminated from your diet, then drinking in moderation is best. If you *do* find that your pain improves when alcohol is eliminated, you would do well to avoid alcohol completely.

Remember that alcoholic beverages also contain a lot of calories. One and a half ounces of gin, rum, vodka, or whiskey contain about 116 calories. A 12-ounce can of beer has about 145 calories.

Using alcohol to numb pain can be problematic. Although it is an age-old analgesic for acute pain, its use in chronic pain can potentially create even more physical and social problems in the long run. Alcohol ingestion within two hours of bedtime can disrupt sleep by reducing deep sleep and dreaming stages. Excessive drinking can also result in liver, pancreas, muscle, and brain dysfunction in susceptible individuals. If you have ever felt that you should cut down on your drinking, been annoyed by people criticizing your drinking, ever felt bad or guilty about your drinking, or ever had a drink first thing in the morning to steady your nerves or get rid of a hangover, then it would be wise to take heed and seek medical help.

MSG. MSG is a flavor enhancer found in many prepared foods but commonly associated with Chinese food. Individuals sensitive to MSG may experience headaches, a burning sensation in the face, sweating, and chest tightness. Studies show that people who experience migraines may or may not be more prone to headaches caused by MSG. Avoidance is the best treatment if you are sensitive. But beware: MSG can be hidden in broth or bouillon cubes and other food products, so read labels to determine whether it is present.

Aspartame. Aspartame (brand name: NutraSweet®) has been associated with headache symptoms in sensitive individuals. Aspartame can be found in a wide assortment of diet products; again, check the labels. If you are drinking a lot of diet drinks or eating a lot of diet products that contain aspartame, you may want to stop consuming them to see whether there is any effect on your pain, especially if you are experiencing headaches.

The Role of Vitamins and Minerals in Reducing Pain

Finally, let's take a look at the role of vitamins and minerals in reducing chronic pain conditions.

The use of magnesium, zinc, B vitamins, and vitamins E and C has been promoted in chronic pain conditions that have an inflammatory component. The lack of consistent scientific findings may reflect human variability and the subjective nature of the pain experience rather than the failure of these supplements to help selected individuals. On the other hand, the lack of consistent positive benefits may indicate that these supplements are of no value. At this time, there is no consistent evidence that ingestion of most mineral or vitamin supplements in addition to your normal diet is helpful in relieving pain. A calcium-rich diet or calcium supplementation is important, however, because of the high incidence of osteoporosis (brittle bones) in postmenopausal women. Vitamin D is also important because of its role in bone formation, but adequate amounts of this vitamin can usually be obtained through milk or exposure to sunlight. Osteoporosis is the number one cause of disability in women over 65 years of age in the United States and is associated with fractures of the spine and hip. Men and women both start losing calcium from their bone stores in their 30s; after menopause, however, the rate of loss for susceptible women is accelerated. Risk factors include the following:

- Having a family history of osteoporosis
- Being a caucasian of northern European background
- Smoking
- Being thin
- Being inactive

There has been a lot of controversy regarding how much and in what form women should take calcium. We know that after menopause there is a need for estrogen replacement before the calcium can be incorporated into bone. For prevention, current recommendations encourage women to get an adequate amount of calcium in their diet before menopause.

The dosage recommended is 1,000 milligrams per day of calcium for nonpregnant, nonlactating women over 25 years of age. This dosage is equal to four eight-ounce glasses of milk or five Tums® tablets a day. For postmenopausal women who are at risk for osteoporosis, the recommended dosage is 1,200–1,500 milligrams of calcium per day, plus estrogen replacement therapy. Other sources of calcium are yogurt, dairy products, and green leafy vegetables. Regular exercise also helps with prevention. There are also medications available to treat osteoporosis, for example, Fosamax®, Miacalcin®, and Evista®.

Summary

Why Discuss Nutrition?

- A chapter on nutrition is included in this book for three reasons: Good nutritional habits are essential for good health; some specific nutritional behaviors can affect pain levels; and there is a lot of misinformation at present about nutritional therapies for pain.
- Studies of nutritional therapies are difficult to carry out for a number of reasons, and the results of such studies must be evaluated with extreme care.
- You can follow some basic nutritional recommendations now to improve your general health and help you in pain management.

Fresh Is Best; Moderation

- The more foods are prepared by others before they reach us, the more likely they are to have added salt, sugar, saturated fats, preservatives, and artificial color.
- Consuming a diet high in fat and sodium and low in fiber can put an individual at risk for developing heart disease, some cancers (colon), high blood pressure, and obesity.
- Eating fresh foods in moderation will help you maintain a stable weight that is appropriate for your height.

Basic Nutritional Guidelines

- The four basic food groups are:
  - Fruits and vegetables
  - Whole grain products, cereals, and breads
  - Low-fat dairy products
  - Lean meat, poultry, fish and other meat substitutes (e.g., beans or legumes, soybean curd, or tofu, and eggs)

- Healthy adults are advised to eat the following daily (these are minimum recommendations; special groups may have different needs):

  - Eat a variety of fruits, vegetables, whole grains, legumes (beans), fish, lean meat, and poultry.
  - Each day eat five servings of vegetables and fruits and six servings of grain products (including whole grains). Eat two servings of a fatty fish per week.
  - Use fat-free and low-fat dairy products.

- The four basic food groups provide us with our requirements of the following nutrients: carbohydrates, proteins, fats, and vitamins and minerals.

Managing Pain through Nutrition

- Try keeping a food diary (see sample at end of book) for several weeks to help you identify how, when, what, and why you eat, as well as to determine any diet-associated patterns in your pain.
- Take time to prepare yourself for eating. Try to eat without distractions, and pay attention to the nourishment you are taking into your body. Take some time after eating to sit quietly and let the food digest.
- Follow these "dos and don'ts" regarding when to eat:

  - Do eat breakfast to get energy for your daily activities.
  - If you suffer from hypoglycemia, do not fast for prolonged periods, and avoid eating sweets as snacks.
  - Don't skip meals.
  - Don't eat most of your calories in the evening.

- Identifying what you eat and any improvement or in negative effect on your pain condition can help you determine which foods to avoid and which foods to keep in your diet.
- Likewise, identifying why you eat can help you establish a relationship between psychological motives for eating (making you feel "better") and the real need for nourishment.
- Experiment with avoiding the following substances if you experience certain symptoms:

  - Caffeine (general pain, stress)
  - Alcohol (migraines or other headaches, general pain)
  - MSG (headaches, burning in face, sweating, chest tightness)
  - Aspartame (headaches)

- At this time there is no consistent evidence that ingestion of most vitamin or mineral supplements in addition to your normal diet is helpful in relieving pain. Calcium supplementation needs to be considered, however, because of the increased incidence of osteoporosis in postmenopausal women and the associated problems due to fractures.

Exploration Tasks

1. Record everything you eat and drink for one week, using the food diary provided at the back of this book. At the end of the week, look your diary over and see where you might like to alter your diet.

   Or for two to four weeks eat a diet with meat substitutes; lots of fruits, grains, and vegetables; no sweet snacks; and no alcohol or caffeine. If you are a big caffeine drinker, you may want to just decrease the total amount of caffeine you drink so you won't suffer any withdrawal symptoms. Observe whether your pain is affected by the dietary change. If you sense any improvement, continue the diet for at least two months to give it a sufficient trial.

2. Set a goal that you want to accomplish related to your diet. Once again, make sure your goal is a behavioral task that you can measure in terms of the steps that *you* will take to accomplish it. Here is an example:

Goal: *Eat five servings of fruits and vegetables a day.*

Steps to take to reach that goal:

A. *List fruits and vegetables that I like.*

B. *Keep track of my intake of food and drink for a week.*

C. *Count up the number of servings of fruits and vegetables I eat a day.*

Now it's your turn.

Goal: _____

Steps to take to reach that goal:

A. _____

B. _____

C. _____

D. _____

In addition, list contingency plans. That is, identify what obstacles might get in the way of your accomplishing this goal. What solutions can you devise to work toward insuring the success of this goal?

	Obstacles	**Solutions**
A.	_____	_____
B.	_____	_____
C.	_____	_____
D.	_____	_____

3. Continue sharing your pleasurable activities. What kind of things have you enjoyed recently? _____

_____

4. What physical exercises have you been able to do on a regular basis? _____

_____

5. If some aspect of changing your nutritional habits (or any other aspect of working with your pain) is causing you particular stress or anxiety, try imagining yourself in a safe, pleasant place (see Chapter 3, RR Technique 5). Describe your special place:

_____

_____

_____

Supplementary Reading

The following books and articles provide additional information on basic nutrition and on nutrition and pain:

American Heart Association, *American Heart Association Low-Fat, Low Cholesterol Cookbook: Heart Healthy, Easy to Make Recipes That Taste Great* (New York: Times Books, 1998).

Gail Darlington and Linda Gamlin, *Diet and Arthritis* (N. Pomfret, VT: Trafalgar Square, 1998).

L. Gail Darlington, "Dietary Therapy for Arthritis," *Rheumatic Disease Clinics of North America, 17*: 273–285, 1991).

Johanna Dwyer, "Nutritional Remedies: Reasonable and Questionable," *Annals of Behavioral Medicine, 14*: 120–125, 1992.

Jens Kjeldsen-Kragh et al., "Controlled Trial of Fasting and One-Year Vegetarian Diet in Rheumatoid Arthritis," *Lancet, 338*: 899–902, 1991.

J. M. Kremer et al., "Effects of High Dose Fish Oil on Rheumatoid Arthritis After Stopping Nonsteroidal Anti-inflammatory Drugs: Clinical and Immune Correlates," *Arthritis and Rheumatology, 38*: 1107–1114, 1995.

D. C. Nordstrom et al., "Alpha Linoleic Acid in the Treatment of Rheumatoid Arthritis: A Double Blind, Placebo Controlled and Randomized Study: Flaxseed vs. Safflower Oil," *Rheumatology International, 14*: 231–234, 1995).

Nutrition Action Health Letter. For subscription information, write to the Center for Science in the Public Interest, 1875 Connecticut Ave. N.W., Suite 300, Washington, DC 20009-5728; or call (202) 332-9110, fax (202) 265-4954, *cspi@cspinet.org*, http://www.cspinet.org.

Richard Panush, "Does Food Cause or Cure Arthritis?" *Rheumatic Disease Clinics of North America, 17*: 259–272, 1991.

Jean A. T. Pennington and Helen Nichols Church, *Bowes and Church's Food Values of Portions Commonly Used*, 13th Edition. (New York: Harper & Row, 1980).

Cynthia Radnitz, "Food Triggered Migraine: A Critical Review," *Annals of Behavioral Medicine, 12*: 51–64, 1990.

Tufts University Diet and Nutrition Letter. For subscription information, write to P.O. Box 420235, Palm Coast, FL 32142; or call (800) 274-7581.

Tufts University Nutrition Navigator. http://navigator.tufts.edu.

Hope S. Warshaw and George Blackburn, *The Restaurant Companion: A Guide to Healthier Eating Out* (Chicago: Surrey Books, 1995).

Andrew Weil, *Eating Well for Optimum Health: The Essential Guide to Food, Diet, and Nutrition* (New York: Knopf, 2000).

Chapter 8

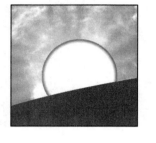

Effective Communication

If you loved me, you'd know what I mean.
—*Me, to my husband*

Communication is a learned set of skills that enables you to get a message across, to express how you feel, to receive feedback, and to listen without judging. The reason a chapter on basic communication skills is included in a book on managing chronic pain is this: Pain patients experience much distress as a result not only of their pain but also of trying to communicate with others about their pain.

There are three basic types of communication problems. Most people, with or without pain, experience these problems at some point:

1. There is a mismatch between the words people speak (their statements) and what they really want (their intentions).
2. People do not state clearly how they feel, what they want, or what they need (assertiveness). They tend either to deny their own feelings ("You count, I don't"—passiveness) or to disregard the feelings of others ("I count, you don't"—aggressiveness).
3. People hear, but they don't really *listen* (active listening).

This chapter describes all three types of problems and provides suggestions for overcoming them.

Making Statements Match Intentions

General Communication: A Sample Scenario

Let's take a look at the following scenario:

> You just came back from shopping, having bought a dress for slightly more money than you would normally spend. This was a treat for participating in the pain program, so you feel only slightly guilty. You put the dress on for dinner that night.
>
> When your husband comes home, you ignore, at first, his observation that the trash barrels have not been brought in. Finally you say, "Well, what do you think?" (You realize that this is a loaded question, given the expense of the dress.)
>
> "About the trash barrels?" he says, only slightly bewildered.
>
> "The dress, the dress!" you exclaim.
>
> "It's okay," he mumbles, really confused now.
>
> You storm out of the room screaming about how insensitive and self-centered he is. You feel that if he loved you, he would know what you meant and want. He is thoroughly baffled.

The first principle of effective communication is to be clear about what you intend in your statements to others. (Although I confess I act at times as if my spouse is a mind reader, it really does not help communication with him or anyone else.) Matching statements with intentions is an art and a skill. It also requires you to assume a certain level of responsibility for your side of the conversation.

Let's go back to the scenario you just read. If your intention is to get positive feedback on your choice in dresses, the fact that you deserve it, and the fact that you look great, you could play Twenty Questions. Or you could say something like this: "I bought myself a dress today as a 'pick-me-up.' I'm looking for confirmation that I chose wisely, that I deserve to treat myself to this, and that you think I look great."

Now there are those who feel that "it doesn't count" if responses don't come spontaneously from the other person. I have not said that the other person (e.g., the husband in the scenario above) is obligated to respond in the way you wish. However, I would venture to say that what you are asking for will be a lot clearer to the other party if your statement reflects your intent. He or she will still be left with the option to comply with your wishes or not.

Communication with Health Care Professionals: Put It in Writing

The following practice exercise may be useful in clarifying your interactions with health care professionals, which can often be both confusing and frustrating because of the mismatch of statements and intentions. It will also serve as a model with which to explore other potential communication conflicts. Do not read further until you've done this exercise.

1. Assume that your pain has become worse. You go to the doctor. What do you say? Write out a statement to your physician. (It is important that you make this an *imaginary* interaction, not one that has actually occurred between you and your physician.)

   _____

   _____

   _____

   _____

2. Now, write what you want the doctor to say back to you.

   _____

   _____

   _____

   _____

In many of our interactions with others, we wish to receive the following:

- Information
- Analysis
- Advice
- Understanding
- Reassurance

If you have completed the exercise above, you will be able to see what it was you wanted by looking at the doctor's statement to you. What were you asking for? Information, advice, analysis, reassurance, understanding, or some combination of these?

If you are like most people, your imaginary statement to the doctor was something like this: "My pain is worse—I hurt more now than ever." End of sentence! If your imaginary "doctor's response" indicated that what you wanted (i.e., your intention) was to receive some advice, analysis, and reassurance, then you may be in for disappointment in real life if the doctor says, "It's nothing. Take two aspirin and call me in the morning."

Try rewriting your first statement to your doctor. This time, however, include clear requests for advice, analysis, information, understanding, and/or reassurance. Here is an example: "My pain is worse. I would like you to examine me and run the appropriate tests to see if this is just a flare-up or something new. Should I change anything in terms of treatment? I'm scared, so I would appreciate it if you would do this to reassure me."

A lot of people find that asking for advice, analysis, or information is easy compared with asking for understanding or reassurance. Sometimes it's because they expect the latter to be automatic: "If you cared about me, you'd know what I want." It may also have to do with the feeling that they are undeserving of this kind of attention or respect.

Doing this exercise can also uncover a "secret" desire for a cure or a miracle. If you are looking for miracles, be up front about it and ask directly. Then you and your physician can at least discuss the newest treatments or lack of them.

If Deborah Tannen, author of *You Just Don't Understand* (see "Supplementary Reading"), is correct that giving advice is a common male communication response, then this may explain why many women patients complain that they do not get statements of reassurance or understanding from the predominantly male medical profession. In fact, women may not even think to ask for such statements. Many medical doctors simply do not feel that statements of reassurance and understanding are relevant in standard communication exchanges; others feel that by giving advice or sharing information, they are demonstrating their understanding or reassurance.

Clearly, if you do not feel the need for reassurance, understanding, or any other item on the list above, then you do not need to ask for it. You are seeking clarification of your unique agenda. If your intentions are unclearly or indirectly stated, you will not get what you need and will feel misunderstood, used, and abused. Of course, just making it clear what you want does not guarantee that you will get it. But I believe you will be pleasantly surprised at the results once you begin practicing clearer communication.

Here are other suggestions for enhancing your interactions with health care professionals. Before your next visit, do the following:

1. Write down your questions, listing the most important ones first.
2. Be ready to describe the symptom or problem that has brought you to the doctor. Keep the description simple and brief.
3. Ask yourself these questions about your symptoms or problem:

   Where is it located?
   When did it start? When does it occur?
   Describe the sensation (symptom): Is it sharp, burning, throbbing, aching, or the like?
   What makes it better?
   What makes it worse?

What have you done about it?

Write down your answers to these questions and bring them with you. Many diagnoses are made from the patterns and interactions of symptoms, so this is important information. You may find it helpful to bring a chart of your pain levels (or symptom patterns).

4. Know what medications you are taking and the dosage for each. Write them down on a card and keep it in your wallet or purse at all times.

5. If you feel that there is a particular issue you need to discuss in detail that requires more than a 15-minute appointment, state this when you call your health care professional. The receptionist is not a mind reader, either.

6. Clarify your expectations. During your visit, are you looking for a miracle, a diagnosis, a treatment plan, or a prognosis?

The Weekly Feedback Sheet provided at the end of this book can also help you to communicate clearly and explicitly with health care professionals.

Assertiveness

"Assertiveness" is a way of expressing how you feel, while respecting the rights of others: "I count, you count." There are three common obstacles to becoming assertive:

1. You do not feel entitled to speak up for how you feel, what you want, or what you need.

2. You confuse assertiveness with passiveness ("You count, I don't") or with aggression ("I count, you don't").

3. You don't know why you feel the way you do, either because you never thought about it or because you are communicating in a style that is based on past assumptions or attitudes.

Obstacle 1: Not Feeling Entitled to Speak Up

Just as you learn irrational beliefs and cognitive distortions, you learn certain "rules" of communication early in life:

"It's not proper to speak unless spoken to."

"Children should be seen and not heard."

"You are obligated to answer all inquiries. If questioned, you can't say 'I don't know.' "

"You should always accommodate others. It's not right to say no."

From these subtle "golden rules," you learn to suppress your opinion. Again, according to Deborah Tannen (see "Supplementary Reading"), you have learned this particularly thoroughly if you are a woman: Females receive different messages about communicating than males do, and one of these is that women should not speak up for themselves.

Many of you may still feel uncomfortable about speaking up for what you feel, want, or need. You may find it helpful to consider assertiveness as a two-way street. You do have a right to express your opinion about how you feel and what you want or think you need; however, there are responsibilities that go along with those rights, which imply your awareness of the rights, wants, and needs of others. Melodie Chenevert, a nurse, writes about the need for rights and responsibilities in her book *Special Techniques in Assertiveness Training: STAT*:

Rights–Responsibilities

Rights	Responsibilities
To speak up	To listen
To take	To give
To have problems	To find solutions
To be comforted	To comfort others
To work	To do your best
To make mistakes	To correct your mistakes
To laugh	To make others happy
To have friends	To be a friend
To criticize	To praise
To have your efforts rewarded	To reward others' efforts
To independence	To be dependable
To cry	To dry tears
To be loved	To love others

From Melodie Chenevert, *Special Techniques in Assertiveness Training: STAT* (St. Louis: C. V. Mosby, 1988, p. 64). Copyright 1988 by C. V. Mosby. Reprinted by permission.

Take time to add other rights and responsibilities to those listed here. The assertive person knows that abusing either rights or responsibilities is self-destructive.

Obstacle 2: Confusing Assertiveness with Passiveness or Aggression

Let's consider three basic styles of interpersonal behavior—passive, aggressive, and assertive—from the perspective of our previous discussion. What are the intentions of passive, aggressive, and assertive statements?

Statement	Intention

Passive

"Okay, whatever you say, I don't care." "Do whatever you want to do [sigh]."	To keep the peace, I don't make waves; I compromise even when it is not called for. You count, I don't.

Aggressive

"You are a jerk! It's all your fault." "I don't care what you say." "You'll do what I say."	To win, I punish, blame, or strike back whenever I think it is necessary. I count, you don't.

Assertive

"I feel sad when you don't ask what I would like to do, because it makes me think you don't care about what I would like or about me. I want you to ask me what I would like to do, and I will promise to come up with some ideas or not hold you responsible if I don't."	I express my feelings, define the behavior that gives rise to those feelings, and state the reason I feel the way I do. Adding "I want" and "I will" expands the assertive statement by clarifying a described action of behavior and identifying my responsibility in this interaction. I count, you count.

The advantage of speaking assertively is that it gives you the opportunity to express your point of view. However, this style also demands a certain honesty about, and a clear understanding of, what it is you really want. Hence, the third obstacle to assertiveness.

Obstacle 3: Not Knowing Why You Feel the Way You Do

What do you want? Why do you want it?

The "formula" for assertive communication is as follows:

"I feel _____ when you _____ because _____."

This formula requires that *all three* elements be included. Many people get stuck after "I feel"; completing the rest of the sentence means getting in touch with yourself and exploring your inner feelings. Let's take a look at why it's important to do so.

> Paul had suffered a painful diabetic neuropathy involving his hands and lower extremities for almost two years and had become unable to do his job as a plumber. Out of work for six months, he found himself bored and irritable.
>
> One day his oldest child came home from school and made the comment that it was cold in the house. Paul became enraged and stormed out to the garage,

where he commonly retreated when he became upset. He said to himself, "It didn't feel cold to me, the child must be a wimp." Upon further reflection, however, he found himself making statements like, "It's the father's responsibility to provide warmth, food, and protection to his family. If I can't provide for my family, then I'm worthless."

Paul had not been aware until then about how distressed he had felt not being able to work. He went back into the house, and after dinner discussed his feelings with his family. His oldest child informed him that the pilot light had gone out on the gas furnace and that he had relit it. They all had a good laugh when Paul told them how angry he had felt when the son had commented about the heat, and how he had taken it as a sign that he couldn't even provide his family with the basics, such as warmth.

Once Paul was able to express his concerns in an assertive way, he was able to receive the reassurance from his family that they understood and did not think him any less of a father or provider because he was not working outside the home.

Theresa, another patient, expressed frustration over a bathroom remodeling project that was going on at home. She found herself extremely irritated with her husband when he showed her a set of faucets that he thought might look nice in the bathroom. She was outraged and responded that the faucets would be hard to clean and that she was the one who would be cleaning them.

When Theresa was asked to turn her response into an assertive statement to her husband, she said, "I feel annoyed when you show me fancy faucets to put in the bathroom, because for the past 25 years you have never taken what I do into consideration. You always take me for granted." She was deluged with and surprised by feelings resulting from 25 years of marital frustrations. An important thing to keep in mind about assertive messages is that they cannot be used to correct all past damages and unspoken hurts. Theresa was able to see this, and realized that her responsibility was to decide what she really wanted to communicate. She also realized that she and her husband needed to do much more talking and be less silent with each other.

Theresa's statement then became this: "I feel conflicted when you ask for my approval of fancy faucets, because, while they are very pretty, I would find them hard to clean. When you present me with what seem to be thoughtless choices, I wonder if you ever think about all that I do at home when you're at work." Actually, as it turned out, her husband had never thought of it that way. He was able to appreciate why she might not be ecstatic about his choice of faucets, and Theresa was able to feel proud that she had stood up for herself.

"I want" statements will help direct the action you feel is desirable. For those situations in which there is a need for compromise or clarification, "I will" statements can facilitate acceptance of the requested action. For example, Theresa might have stated to her husband, "If you bring me a catalogue of faucets, I will make an effort to choose one that suits my needs."

It's important to differentiate between a hurtful and aggressive statement and one that is used to clarify your feelings or intentions. For example, the statement "I feel you are a jerk" is not assertive, even though it begins with "I feel." Although aggressive statements may flow more easily than assertive ones, they rarely accomplish anything except revenge ("I showed them"), which is usually short-lived. They either complicate further communication possibilities or eliminate them altogether.

Passive statements, such as "It's up to you" or "I don't care," may be appropriate at times when used judiciously and consciously. If they merely reinforce martyrdom or self-abuse, then they too will poison communication attempts and relationships.

The major difficulties in beginning assertive communication are (1) becoming conscious of why you feel the way you do; and (2) taking responsibility for how you feel, rather than blaming others or wishing things could be different. One of the reasons that Chapter 5 gives you the opportunity to identify negative self-talk and other negative responses is to help you overcome these difficulties. Although at first it may seem uncomfortable or awkward to state directly how you feel, it allows for true dialogue (two-way communication) to take place. Completing the Assertiveness Questionnaire, provided at the end of this chapter, will enable you to identify the situations in which assertiveness may be more awkward for you.

Active Listening

Active listening is a technique that, when practiced with conscious awareness, can de-escalate (or at least clarify the issues involved in) many emotional interchanges. It is a first step in conflict resolution and prevention. Active listening requires hearing—*not* judging, parroting, questioning, supporting, rationalizing, or defending—what someone else is saying.

For example, suppose that your spouse announces, "I'm fed up with how messy the house always looks." Now this is understandably a loaded statement, because you may already be feeling uneasy about your inability to keep things tidy with your pain problem. Here are some unhelpful possible replies:

- *Judging*: "You shouldn't feel that way."
- *Parroting*: "So you feel the house is always messy."
- *Questioning*: "Really? Do you have any brilliant ideas on how to keep it clean?"
- *Supporting*: "Things will get better. I'll try harder."
- *Rationalizing*: "You've had a hard day at work. Sit down and cool off."
- *Defending*: "I do the best I can, but you're never satisfied."

Some of these statements sound more reasonable than others, but each one ends the discussion prematurely—either by jumping to conclusions, by disallowing further information, or by putting off conversation.

A phrase that may be useful in cases such as this one comes from the work of psychologist Carl Rogers:

"You sound _____ about _____."

Let's fill in the blanks to explore the scenario further: "You sound *upset* about *the messy house.*" Possible responses from your spouse include the following:

"Oh, it's not just the clutter here, it's the clutter at work. I feel so overwhelmed because I can't get things done. I have two projects due. . . . "

"You better believe I'm upset. I work hard all day and I don't like coming home to a house in disarray."

With active listening, you buy time and get a better idea of what the other person is feeling. Then you can make a choice between expending the energy or effort to answer, or deciding not to involve yourself in the other person's distress at the time.

Once the other person has responded, and you have decided to reply, learning to deflect responses that are potential sources of conflict can be very rewarding. Acknowledging how the other person feels permits both parties to respect their differences; clarifying the actual source of distress facilitates discussion and problem solving on neutral ground. For example, a possible reply to the response, "You better believe I'm upset. . . . " might be the following: "I'm sorry you're upset. I wanted to check out whether it was me, the messy house, or something else that was bothering you." From here, the conversation could proceed to problem solving—that is, how to handle the fact that the house is messy and that it may be difficult to keep it clean.

Active listening thus serves to diffuse emotional energies that could quickly escalate into confrontation. It also allows you to be reflective, empathic, objective, and nonjudgmental. By identifying the feeling that you are perceiving, you are encouraging the other person to express himself or herself further. And by clarifying to whom or to what these feelings are being directed, you are promoting problem solving and reinforcing a healthier expression of emotions. Like any new behavior, active listening takes practice—but it is well worth the effort.

Further Suggestions for Communication Practice

Perhaps people have a difficult time changing their communication styles because communication is something they think little about once they have learned to speak. Some suggestions, however, may facilitate your practice. In the beginning, as with monitoring your self-talk, the process appears long and laborious. After a while, however, you find yourself examining your self-talk whenever negative physical or emotional cues are perceived. Likewise, when you experience an interpersonal conflict or discomfort, it is a good time to pause and reflect on what or where the communication problem might be. Has your intent been clearly stated? Are you being passive or aggressive out of habit? Have you considered where the other person is coming from, or have you simply assumed you knew? Is it a gender-based or cultural conflict that involves styles, not personality issues?

To illustrate the last of these points, I was once on a trip with a group of Spanish, English, and American tourists. We stopped in a small Greek resort town to eat lunch. After we had waited in the buffet line for over an hour, the problem became apparent. We overheard various English and Spanish groups discussing it with great animation. Each nationality was accusing the other of "queuing up" (i.e., lining up) from the "wrong" side. The English claimed that "everyone knows that you queue from the left"; the Spanish were just as vehement about queuing from the right. (The Americans, of course, just barged right into the middle of the line.) The conflict, which quickly became personalized, was based on cultural factors that no group was willing or able to acknowledge at the time. Major battles have probably been started over misunderstandings of even lesser magnitude and significance.

Taking responsibility for our words and thoughts is not easy. We tend automatically to apply long-term attitudes (ones we have not consciously considered recently, if at all) to short-term problems. On the other hand, because we tend to be short-sighted as humans, our solutions are focused on quick fixes and immediate gratifications. Few of us can afford to indulge in these ways of thinking. As you will see for yourself, practicing effective communication skills as presented in this chapter does facilitate deserved and necessary dialogue with the outside world.

Summary

- There are three important aspects of communication: making statements match intentions; assertiveness; and active listening.
- Making statements match intentions refers to being clear in your original statement about what it is you really mean. It is particularly important in communication with health care providers, in which you should make it plain whether you are requesting information, analysis, advice, understanding, and/or reassurance.
- Assertiveness is a positive and direct way of expressing how you feel while respecting the rights of others. There are three common obstacles to becoming assertive:

  - Not feeling entitled to speak up
  - Confusing assertiveness with passiveness or aggression
  - Not knowing why you feel the way you do

- Active listening is a conscious technique; it requires hearing what someone else is saying without assuming that you know what the person is trying to say.

Exploration Tasks

1. Complete the Assertiveness Questionnaire, provided at the end of this chapter. What did you learn?

   _____

   _____

   _____

   How might you more effectively manage those situations in which assertiveness is a problem for you?

   _____

   _____

   _____

   _____

2. Identify an assertive communication: As you go through your week, be aware of any difficult conversations—situations in which you either spoke assertively or did not but should have. Write down the key elements of the dialogue in one conversation.

   I said: _____

   _____

   _____

   The other person said: _____

   _____

   _____

   I said: _____

   _____

   _____

   He or she said: _____

   _____

   _____

   I said: _____

   _____

   _____

   Once you have recorded the conversation, analyze it in terms of the assertive communication guidelines discussed in this chapter. Did you use "I" sentences ("I feel," "I want," etc.)? Did you describe the specific behavior that was troubling you and why? Did you express your opinion and views and respect those of the other person?

Finally, look at what followed the conversation. If you were assertive, what stress do you think you avoided? If you were not assertive, what stress did you create for yourself?

3. Continue to keep track of your negative self-talk and other negative responses, using the worksheet provided at the end of the book for this purpose. Now, consider this question: How can you reframe those thoughts to reflect the reality of the situation, using "I can" and "I need" statements? Pay particular attention to those situations involving conflict in communication with others. What is the source of the conflict as you see it? Are there unspoken assumptions or expectations involved? Do you have the "whole picture," or do you need more information?

4. Practice the "You sound _____ about _____" listening response to the following statements, and then use an assertive response ("I feel _____ when you _____ because _____") to practice stating your intent. Use the "I want" and "I will" statements, too.

A. "You should be better by now! There is nothing wrong on X-rays or blood tests, and yet you still have pain. I have nothing more to offer you!"

Listening response: _____

_____

_____

Assertive response: _____

_____

_____

B. "Every time I call you to do something, you give me this vague story about not knowing if you'll be able to go."

Listening response: _____

_____

_____

Assertive response: _____

_____

_____

C. "What is this, a perpetual vacation? When are you going back to work, or are you not going to give up a good thing?"

Listening response: _____

_____

_____

Assertive response: _____

_____

_____

5. Write out a goal that you want to accomplish related to the material in this chapter. As always, make sure your goal is a behavioral task that you can measure in terms of the steps *you* will take to accomplish it. Here is an example:

Goal: *To practice clear communication with my doctor at my next visit.*

Steps to take to reach that goal:

A. *Clarify my expectations of the visit by writing out a statement to the doctor. Make sure it reflects my intentions.*

B. *Chart my pain on a graph so that the preceding four-week pattern is displayed.*

C. *Bring my medication list with me.*

D. *Write out my questions before I go, putting the most important ones first.*

Now it's your turn.

Goal: _____

Steps to take to reach that goal:

A. _____

B. _____

C. _____

D. _____

In addition, list contingency plans. That is, identify what obstacles might get in the way of your accomplishing this goal. What solutions can you devise to work toward insuring the success of this goal?

	Obstacles	**Solutions**
A.	_____	_____
B.	_____	_____
C.	_____	_____
D.	_____	_____

6. Now is a good time to start exploring RR Technique 7 (see Chapter 3), if you have not already tried it. After you have worked with the pain image, you can put other problems behind the clear plastic wall to examine. This distancing yourself from a problem can help you develop an objective view of the issue and perhaps become more effective at problem solving.

Supplementary Reading

The following books provide additional information on communication skills:

David Burns, *The Feeling Good Handbook* (New York: Plume, 1999).

David Burns, *Ten Days to Self-Esteem* (New York: Quill/William Morrow, 1999).

Martha Davis, Elizabeth Robbins Eshelman, and Matthew McKay, *The Relaxation and Stress Reduction Workbook* (Oakland, CA: New Harbinger, 2000).

Roger Fisher and William Ury, *Getting to Yes: Negotiating Agreement without Giving In* (New York: Penguin, 1991).

Jenny Steinmetz, Jon Blankenship, Linda Brown, Deborah Hall, and Grace Miller, *Managing Stress Before It Manages You* (Palo Alto, CA: Bull, 1980).

Deborah Tannen, *That's Not What I Meant! How Conversational Style Makes or Breaks Relationships* (New York: Ballantine Books, 1991).

Deborah Tannen, *You Just Don't Understand: Women and Men in Conversation* (New York: Ballantine Books, 1991).

Assertiveness Questionnaire

To further refine your assessment of the situations in which you need to be more assertive, complete the following questionnaire. Put a check mark in column A by the items that are applicable to you and then rate those items in column B as:

1. Comfortable
2. Mildly uncomfortable
3. Moderately uncomfortable
4. Very uncomfortable
5. Unbearably threatening

(Note that the varying degrees of discomfort can be expressed whether your inappropriate reactions are hostile or passive.)

A Check here if the item applies to you	B Rate from 1–5 for discomfort	*When* do you behave nonassertively?
_____	_____	Asking for help
_____	_____	Stating a difference of opinion
_____	_____	Receiving and expressing negative feelings
_____	_____	Receiving and expressing positive feelings
_____	_____	Dealing with someone who refuses to cooperate
_____	_____	Speaking up about something that annoys you
_____	_____	Talking when all eyes are on you
_____	_____	Protesting a rip-off
_____	_____	Saying "No"
_____	_____	Responding to undeserved criticism
_____	_____	Making requests of authority figures
_____	_____	Negotiating for something you want
_____	_____	Having to take charge
_____	_____	Asking for cooperation
_____	_____	Proposing an idea
_____	_____	Taking charge
_____	_____	Asking questions

(*cont.*)

A Check here if the item applies to you	B Rate from 1–5 for discomfort	*When* do you behave nonassertively?
_____	_____	Dealing with attempts to make you feel guilty
_____	_____	Asking for service
_____	_____	Asking for a date or appointment
_____	_____	Asking for favors
_____	_____	Other: _____

A Check here if the item applies to you	B Rate from 1–5 for discomfort	*Who* are the people with whom you are nonassertive?
_____	_____	Parents
_____	_____	Fellow workers or classmates
_____	_____	Strangers
_____	_____	Old friends
_____	_____	Spouse or mate
_____	_____	Employer
_____	_____	Relatives
_____	_____	Children
_____	_____	Acquaintances
_____	_____	Sales people, clerks, hired help
_____	_____	More than two or three people in a group
_____	_____	Other: _____

A Check here if the item applies to you	B Rate from 1–5 for discomfort	*What* do you want that you have been unable to achieve with nonassertive styles?
_____	_____	Approval for things that you have done well
_____	_____	To get help with certain tasks
_____	_____	More attention time with your mate
_____	_____	To be listened to and understood
_____	_____	To make boring or frustrating situations more satisfying
_____	_____	To not have to be nice all the time
_____	_____	Confidence in speaking up when something is important to you

_____	_____	Greater comfort with strangers, store clerks, mechanics, etc.
_____	_____	Confidence in asking for contact with people you find attractive
_____	_____	To get a new job, ask for interviews, raises, and so on
_____	_____	Comfort with people who supervise you or work under you
_____	_____	To not feel angry and bitter a lot of the time
_____	_____	To overcome a feeling of helplessness and the sense that nothing ever really changes
_____	_____	To initiate satisfying sexual experiences
_____	_____	To do something totally different and novel
_____	_____	To have time by yourself
_____	_____	To do things that are fun or relaxing for you
_____	_____	Other: _____

Evaluating Your Responses

Examine your answers, and analyze them for an overall picture of what situations and people are more threatening. How does nonassertive behavior contribute to the specific items you checked on the "What" list? In constructing your own assertiveness program, it will be initially useful to focus on items you rated as falling in the 2–3 range. These are the situations that you will find easiest to change. Items that are very uncomfortable or threatening can be tackled later.

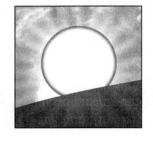

Chapter 9

Effective Problem Solving

The problems that exist in the world cannot be solved by the level of thinking that created them.

—Albert Einstein

People often get caught up in trying to solve problems before they are prepared to do so. Many times in previous chapters, you may have come to a point at which problem solving seemed to be the next logical step. But first you had to be able to quiet your mind chatter through RR techniques; to clarify what you think and feel; to understand how attitudes can affect your ability to cope with stress; and to identify your communication style and improve your communication skills. Problem solving requires setting clear goals; identifying emotional barriers (hooks) that may prevent goals from being accomplished; and identifying the small sequential steps needed to fulfill the goal. Now you are ready to begin problem solving.

Setting Goals: A Closer Look

Take a moment to write down three goals that you would like to accomplish in the next six months. You have been asked to set goals at the end of each chapter, and so the task has probably become less difficult. If you need to refresh your memory on setting goals, however, refer to Chapter 1.

1. Goal: _____

2. Goal: _____

3. Goal: _____

As you may well have discovered, though, accomplishing goals can be considerably more difficult than setting them. Often, failing to accomplish your goals has little or nothing to do with the steps you identify to help you along the way. For example, let's take a look at a goal that was determined by Barbara, a previous patient.

The Emotional Hook

Barbara stated that one of her goals was to go back to work. I asked her why she hadn't done it before this. After some comments relating to her being in pain and not knowing what to do, she suddenly paused. "You know, the truth is ... I'm terrified at the prospect." I asked her to write about the problem—her terror—in the format used to examine the automatic thoughts or self-talk associated with negative emotions:

Situation	Thought	Emotion	Distortion
Going back to work	"I'll never keep up"	Terrified	Jumping to conclusions
	"I'll reinjure myself"	Anxious	Fortune telling

What Barbara was experiencing can be called an "emotional hook." Emotional hooks are the cognitive distortions explored in Chapter 5. Just picture those big vaudeville hooks that pulled bad acts off the stage. An emotional hook consists of self-defeating talk, arising from the cognitive distortions and irrational beliefs that get in the way of accomplishing your goals or block your ability to solve problems.

As long as Barbara remained fearful and anxious about whether she would be able to perform or might get reinjured, her emotional hook would pull her away (like a bad vaudeville act) from effectively solving the problem and reaching her goal (and her show would not go on!). Emotional hooks need to be dealt with before real problem solving can begin. Fortunately, you already have the tools to cope with emotional hooks; they are the same ones you use to deal with negative self-talk. First, identify your feelings, your self-talk, and the cognitive distortions/irrational beliefs behind them. Then challenge the reality of those thoughts.

Barbara challenged the thoughts behind her fear. According to objective tests performed by her occupational health specialist, her pain problem was chronic, and a regular work routine was not going to harm her. She knew that she could ask for reasonable accommodations in the workplace if she was partially disabled or impaired under the Americans with Disabilities Act (see "Supplementary Reading"). She had been practicing alternating pain-increasing activities with pain-decreasing activities for a while and would adjust this to her work routine using the Post-it® Note ideas from Chapter 4. She knew that she would need to continue her exercise, conditioning program, communicate her need for changing positions throughout her workday, and regularly destress herself with mini-relaxations. She was now ready to feel the fear but do it anyway!

Identifying the Barriers to Accomplishing Your Goals

> That which we do not bring to consciousness appears in our life as fate.
> —*Carl Gustav Jung*

Can you identify the emotional hook that might be getting in the way of accomplishing one of your goals? Start by questioning why you haven't achieved your goal yet, or pick a goal you feel will be difficult to achieve. (In many cases, goals that are thought of as difficult harbor emotional hooks.) When you consider this goal, are you aware of feeling anxious, fearful, or overwhelmed? Once you have identified the emotion you feel, put it in the same format that Barbara did above, identifying the self-talk (the hook) and the cognitive distortions that go with it. How will you challenge your thoughts? Now, what is the "problem" that needs solving? Solving the actual problem is often surprisingly easy, once it is untangled from the emotional hook.

Here's an exercise in identifying an emotional hook and then restating the problem:

Write down one of your goals (see what you wrote at the beginning of this chapter) that you feel may be difficult.

Goal: _____

When you think about why you haven't accomplished this goal up to now or why you think it might be difficult, what do you feel? For example: overwhelmed, anxious, fearful.

Feelings (emotional response): _____

What kind of self-talk do you find yourself saying when you think about this emotion or the difficulty of the goal? For example, "I can't do it. What if I fail?"

Self-talk (automatic thoughts) (a.k.a. emotional hook): _____

_____

Next, identify the source of the self-talk in terms of distortions, catastrophizing, avoidance, denial, and irrational beliefs. For example, "I shouldn't have to make changes, it wasn't my fault" = cognitive distortion; "Life should be fair" = irrational belief; "This is the worst thing that could happen and I can't take it" = catastrophizing.

Cognitive distortion or irrational beliefs (Chapter 5)/**Negative attitudes** (Chapter 6):

_____

_____

Now challenge the thoughts that are unrealistic and reflect on the reality of the situation you find yourself in. What can you do and what do you need? If you get stuck, use the Vertical Arrow Technique (see Chapter 5) or write about your problem for 20 minutes and see what comes up. For example: "It's not fair that I have to change how I do things, but this is about going forward, creating a new life with pain. What is required is my changing how I do things."

Challenges to self-talk: _____

_____

_____

How do you feel now about the possibility of accomplishing your goal? Relieved, sad, but committed?

Now you are in a better position to set the steps for achieving your goal because, having faced the source of your goblins and ghouls, you won't sabotage your success!

Identifying the Steps Needed for Goal Achievement

When setting up your goal, particularly if it is an ambitious one, it is important to break it down into the many small steps you will need to take to reach the bigger goal. These steps can be grouped into smaller goals. This will help to guarantee your successful accomplishment of the larger goal.

For example, Barbara's goal was to succeed in her return to work. She was able to break that large goal down into the following smaller steps: She would update her resume, determine what kind of job she wanted and could do, get help from the state's vocational rehabilitation services, and start getting job applications. She would continue to do her exercise routine but split it up between the morning and afternoon or evening to accommodate a work schedule. She would make sure that she had a routine of getting up and going to bed at the same time. She identified friends that she could talk with should she begin to feel overwhelmed and made a commitment to continue attending church weekly to get the spiritual support she needed. She moved her relaxation technique to bedtime to make sure she would go to sleep in the most relaxed state. She identified some cookbooks that could assist her in cooking quick but healthy meals. She checked with her occupational therapist to review other assistive devices that she might incorporate into the performance of her occupational goals. Barbara could now move toward accomplishing her return to work.

Note that the steps for Barbara's goal to succeed on her return to work could be specified and subdivided still further. The more thoroughly you clarify the steps, the more likely you are to accomplish the goal.

Contingency plans are also helpful. First described in the "Exploration Tasks" for Chapter 3, these plans help insure that you can't "lose." Barbara made some contingency plans to make sure that she would achieve her goal of success at work. For example, she made arrangements to stop at the company's health service office at noon if her pain was getting worse, so that she could elicit the RR in a private room. She also arranged for a massage therapist to call if her pain flared up.

Take your goal and break it down into the steps you will need to take to reach it. Be as specific as you can, dividing each step into smaller steps whenever necessary.

1. _____
   A. _____
   B. _____
   C. _____

2. _____
   A. _____
   B. _____
   C. _____

3. _____
   A. _____
   B. _____
   C. _____

4. _____
   A. _____
   B. _____
   C. _____

Now list contingency plans. As in earlier chapters' "Exploration Tasks," remember to define these in terms of possible obstacles and their solutions.

Obstacles	Solutions
_____	_____
_____	_____
_____	_____
_____	_____

Assessing Your Ways of Coping and Applying Them to Problems

If you started at the beginning of this book and have done all the exercises, you have now accumulated a considerable number of ways of coping. To assist you in remembering what you've learned, it may be helpful to categorize the skills in the following way:

- Physical ways of coping
- Emotion-focused coping
- Problem-focused coping

The physical ways of coping include aerobic exercise, labeling your sensations, pacing your activities, RR techniques, and so on. The emotion-focused coping skills include RR techniques, capturing negative self-talk and challenging it, assertiveness, and so forth. The problem-focused coping skills include setting goals, seeking pleasurable activities, identifying resources for obtaining more information, brainstorming with friends and associates, securing social support, and the like.

You will note that a particular skill may fall into more than one category, depending on how it is used and for what purpose. For example, an RR technique can be used to calm a tense body (physical coping), as well as a tense emotional state (emotion-focused coping).

Many times, when people ask friends or relatives for help in solving problems, there is an immediate move to problem solving: "Have you tried this or that?" or "My aunt had that problem and she did this." As you have seen earlier in this chapter, moving to problem solving too early and too quickly can frustrate effective problem solving if there is an emotional hook. Such a hook requires coping with the emotional content. Similarly, people who have used physical ways of coping (e.g., strenuous exercise) to the exclusion of other skills for their stress management find themselves very depressed when physical activity is altered by chronic pain. Having a variety of skills and knowing when to use them in solving problems are essential to managing life in general and life with chronic pain in particular.

As in any program that offers a variety of skills, you probably have found yourself gravitating to some skills more than others. You may also have found some skills more difficult to learn than others. But keep practicing all of them.

Take some time to go back through the book to see whether you can identify all the skills you have learned. Can you organize the skills into the three categories below? Put an asterisk (*) by the ones you still need to work on. Creating a list of your skills will come in handy when we discuss planning for pain flare-ups.

Physical ways of coping: _____

_____

_____

_____

_____

Emotion-focused coping skills: _____

_____

_____

_____

_____

Problem-focused coping skills: _____

_____

_____

_____

_____

_____

The following poem (from Portia Nelson's *There's a Hole in My Sidewalk*; Appendix D, Bibliography) summarizes the self-discovery process—the same process you have begun by reading this book.

An Autobiography in Five Chapters

Chapter 1
   I walk down the street.
   There is a deep hole in the sidewalk. I fall in.
   I am lost. . . . I am helpless. It isn't my fault.
   It takes forever to find a way out.

Chapter 2
   I walk down the same street.
   There is a deep hole in the sidewalk.
   I pretend I don't see it.
   I fall in again.
   I can't believe I am in this same place.
   But it isn't my fault.
   It still takes a long time to get out.

Chapter 3
   I walk down the same street.
   There is a deep hole in the sidewalk.
   I see it is there.
   I fall in . . . it's a habit . . . but my eyes are open.
   I know where I am.
   It is my fault.
   I get out immediately.

Chapter 4
   I walk down the same street.
   There is a deep hole in the sidewalk.
   I walk around it.

Chapter 5
   I walk down a different street.

—Portia Nelson

Summary

- If you are finding a goal difficult to accomplish, do the following:

  - Look for the presence of an emotional hook (negative automatic thoughts or self-defeating talk).
  - Identify the emotional hook and the cognitive distortions that go with it.
  - Challenge and change the self-talk.
  - Now restate the goal.

- Identify the steps you need to take to solve a problem or accomplish a goal; the more thoroughly you break down and clarify the steps, the more likely you are to accomplish the goal. Contingency plans also help insure success.
- Assess and categorize the skills you have learned in this program as follows:

  - Physical ways of coping
  - Emotion-focused coping
  - Problem-focused coping
  - Having a variety of skills and knowing when to use them in solving problems are essential.

Exploration Tasks

1. Of the three goals you wrote at the beginning of this chapter, you have analyzed one in the exercises included in the chapter text. Now analyze the other two goals.

   Goal: _____

   Emotion: _____

   Self-talk (a.k.a. emotional hook): _____

   _____

   Cognitive distortion: _____

   _____

   Challenges to self-talk: _____

   _____

   Other skills you might use to cope with the emotional hook (e.g., assertiveness, RR techniques): (Note that this was *not* part of the original analysis in the chapter text, but respond in terms of what you have learned about the different types of coping skills.)

   _____

   _____

   _____

Steps to take to solve problem or reach goal (be as specific as you can):

A. _____

   • _____

   • _____

   • _____

B. _____

   • _____

   • _____

   • _____

C. _____

   • _____

   • _____

   • _____

D. _____

   • _____

   • _____

   • _____

*   *   *

Goal: _____

Emotion: _____

Self-talk (a.k.a. emotional hook): _____

_____

Cognitive distortion: _____

_____

Challenges to self-talk: _____

_____

Other skills you might use to cope with the emotional hook (e.g., assertiveness, RR techniques): _____

_____

_____

Steps to take to solve problem or reach goal (be as specific as you can):

A. _____

   • _____

   • _____

   • _____

2. Draw a picture of yourself with crayons or colored pencils on the following page. Do not look at your earlier drawing (see Chapter 1) until after you have completed your second drawing. Do you notice any differences? What are they?

Supplementary Reading

Americans with Disabilities Act Handbook, Equal Employment Opportunity Commission and Justice Dept. 1992. Available through Amazon.com and Barnes and Noble; disAbility.gov or http://disability.gov/CSS/Default.asp (resources for employment).

Christopher W. Hoenig, *The Problem Solving Journey: Your Guide to Making Decisions and Getting Results* (Reading, MA: Perseus Books, 2000).

Richard S. Lazarus and Susan Folkman, *Stress, Appraisal, and Coping* (New York: Springer, 1984).

Use this space to draw a picture of yourself.

Chapter 10

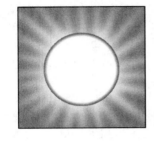

The End of the Beginning

This is not the end. It is not even the beginning of the end. But it is the end of the beginning.

—*Winston Churchill*

A great deal of material has been presented for your consumption in this book. There is no one place at which you are expected to be at this point. Much of the work that you have done will stay with you and grow as your life evolves. Many graduates of the program have told me that it took about six months before they were confident about the changes they had begun. Continued skills practice, periodically reviewing the book, and staying connected with supportive friends and family were all helpful in sustaining the gains they had made. For many, continued learning and reinforcement was made possible by reading the materials listed in the "Supplementary Reading" sections (see also Appendix D).

My own experience with practicing the various skills in this book is that, although life continues to present me with stressors, I have more control in how I respond to those stressors, and that has made all the difference. For almost all who have worked with this program, pain remains a presence. Most of them, however, have established (or at least begun to establish) satisfying and fulfilled lives beyond the pain.

Relapse Prevention

It is important to think ahead during your good periods about how you might handle the more difficult times. This kind of planning ahead is called "relapse prevention." It helps to insure that a relapse either won't occur or will be short-lived if it does occur.

Sometimes, after people have started to use coping skills in managing their pain, they may have a "honeymoon period" in which things aren't so bad. At those times, skills such as pacing or the RR techniques may not be practiced as regularly. Or things may get pretty bad, and they get discouraged again that "nothing will work." And so they give up because of their unrealistic feelings that "it should be better by now." There may be other barriers to continuing with these new behaviors: lack of encouragement from those around you, increased personal stress, increased pain, additional health problems, "time constraints," or "inconvenience." All of these problems have been addressed in this book, but change in behavior is a process of forward steps and periodic retreats. Our research has found that those people with chronic pain who have completed the program and believe they can manage their pain report less depression and less pain and are less disabled. Working with the materials in this book can help you become effective in managing your own pain. That includes anticipating the problems that might confront you and planning ahead now to cope with them.

Make a list of what might get in the way of your continuing with the skills you have learned in this book. List those on the "Problem" line below. Then for each problem, consider how you could get yourself back on track.

Example:

Problem: No one with whom to share the successes and difficulties of living with chronic pain.
Solution: Join a support group, keep a diary of your experiences.

Problem: Loss of a job.
Solution: Reread Chapter 9 on effective problem solving, contact vocational rehabilitation resource.

Problem: _____
Solution: _____

Problem: _____
Solution: _____

Problem: _____
Solution: _____

Coping with Pain during a Flare-Up

When the pain flares up or a crisis occurs, you may forget some of what you have learned. We are all vulnerable to returning to old habits when we are feeling out of control, even if these habits have not served us well in the past. Pain flare-ups are often inevitable and difficult.

In spite of the emphasis in this program on the chronic nature of pain, many people expect that things should be better and that increases in their pain will not occur after their hard work. Needless to say, they are unhappy to find that this is not the case. Because of the complex nature of chronic pain involving mind and body, emotions and sensations, brain and nerves, the normal course of events is for the pain to have periodic increases and decreases that you may or may not be able to predict. Where you have control in such matters is in limiting the distress associated with the pain increase by applying comfort measures that will keep the pain at more tolerable levels and in adjusting your functioning according to the discomfort you feel. Unless a disease or underlying process (nerve damage) has progressed, the great majority of pain flare-ups in chronic pain are short-lived and are just variations in the "volume control" of the pain system.

Coping with the Stages of Pain

There are two ways of approaching the problem of coping with pain flare-ups. One is to write down your plan for routine daily management, for mild to moderate pain increases, and for severe pain increases. Make a copy of this plan and give it to your health care professional. For example:

Daily Management

1. Medication: Gabapentin 300 mg three times a day, amitriptyline 100 mg at bedtime
2. Daily stretching, pool aerobics three times per week
3. Daily RR practice

Mild to Moderate Pain Increase

1. Heat or ice for comfort
2. Transcutaneous nerve stimulator (TENS)
3. Muscle relaxant
4. Call a friend

Severe Pain Increase

1. Reduce activities
2. Watch a favorite movie
3. Increase gabapentin to two 300-mg capsules three times a day for a few days
4. Ice massage

Now it's your turn:

Daily Management

_____

_____

_____

Mild to Moderate Pain Increase

_____

_____

_____

Severe Pain Increase

_____

_____

_____

Panic Plan

Another way of identifying strategies of coping with pain flare-ups is to develop a "panic plan." The idea is that instead of panicking when pain increases, you can refer to a detailed list of things you have identified to be helpful for the mind, body, and spirit. Making this list ahead of time will give you the guidance to take action when you have your pain flare-up. The more specific you make the plan, the easier it will be to follow. For example, if you say "Call a friend," then add a detail such as "Mary Smith's phone number is 888-0983." Or if you say "Relax," add more specific details on how to relax (e.g., "Do breath focusing," "Take a bath with lavender bath salts," or "Watch my favorite sport on TV").

To help you cope with your pain during a flare-up, make a list of the options, skills, and techniques you have. _Be as specific as you can_. Later you'll be able to refer to this list and know exactly what to do without thinking. It's also a good way to reviewing the coping skills you have learned. You don't have to limit your list to your new behavioral techniques: previous steps you have taken to alleviate your discomfort, such as applying ice or heat and using medication, can be included, too.

For my mind . . .

1. RR technique—guided imagery
2. _____
3. _____
4. _____

For my body . . .

1. Hot shower
2. _____
3. _____
4. _____

For my spirit . . .

1. Call my friend John 222-444-5555
2. _____
3. _____
4. _____

Make copies of this list to carry with you, put on your refrigerator door, and/or keep in the glove compartment of your car. In other words, keep the list handy in various places for quick reference.

Now that you've completed your list, refer to the end of Chapter 1, where you were asked to write a similar list of things you did when the pain got worse. Do you find that things have changed?

A Celebration!

This program should end with a celebration. If you are in a group, poems can be read or exchanged, thank-yous expressed to other members, music played, and/or festive food shared.

If you are not in a group, take a moment and close your eyes. Imagine yourself in a room full of people. You realize that these people are strangers, but there is a sense of a common purpose and struggle. The room is vibrant with laughter, smells of food, and animated conversations—conversations about successful pacing of activities, who was assertive with whom, and recent pleasurable activities. Slowly, you realize that these people have just read the same book and worked with the same pain program you have been exploring. By your efforts and hard work, you have become part of a universal group of people who have chosen to take an active role in their pain management. Enjoy your celebration with your imaginary colleagues, or, alternatively, give yourself the opportunity to enjoy the glow of a job well done. Reward yourself by going out to dinner with a friend, treating yourself to a getaway weekend or vacation, buying yourself some flowers, or all of the above!

Here are four examples of poems or other materials shared by program participants; all speak to the struggles, the courage, and the triumphs of individuals in chronic pain. At the end of the chapter, space is provided for *you* to write and express your thoughts to your unseen colleagues. A special thanks to all of you for sharing your experience.

Journey

I do not wish to be
as the log in a hot fire,
burning and raging
against its inevitable
fall to ashes.

I wish to be
as the pebble at an ocean;
washed and molded
by the waves and the sand,
warmed by the sun,
lifted by the tide,
everchanging.

—*S. E. Long*

Given

I will open this gift of pain,
Loosen its cords of rage,
Unfold the wrap of sorrow.

Is it a garment? I shall put it on
And disappear at once from sight.
(How much invisibility can I endure?)

I think it is an iron yoke of discipline,
It rings with authority:
My will must learn its place.

There is more, there is
Admission to another University.
Hard lessons.
Every leaf in the world
Must thirst before it falls.
Each predator becomes another's prey.
The mountain melts, earth labors.
Stars too must burn.
This little pandemonium in my brain
Opens a wide door.
To bear pain is to dance in holy fire
With Shiva the Unmaker
Who turns and turns forever his bright clay.
The gift of pain is knowing,
Knowing: it is so.

—*Margo Harvey*

A Gift from the Wish List

The door to the elevator was being held open for me as I stepped in.

"Thanks," I said before I realized it was he who provided the courtesy. Alone with just our reflections against the polished door, I felt I had to break the awkward silence.

"Excuse me, but don't I . . . "

"Bruce? Well I'll be darned! How are you?"

"Oh, just fine," I lied. "And you?"

I already knew the answer. I had seen him for the last two weeks in my chronic pain management course, but something had kept me from walking right up and saying hello. Maybe I wasn't really sure it was him, it had been so long.

"God, let me look at you!" he said, yanking off my ever-present cap.

"Hair's looking pretty thin," he chided.

"And you've put on a few pounds, I see," I countered. "No wonder I didn't recognize you in class."

The door opened at the ground floor, mercifully ending our mutual embarrassment at acting like strangers for the past two weeks.

"How long has it been?" I asked. "Can it have been fifteen years?"

"Almost twenty," he corrected, staring off as if surprised by his answer himself.

We spent two or three minutes standing there in the lobby, reminiscing about the old days. We were inseparable back then. Raised hell together and shared our secrets with each other. Then came marriage, careers, family. We lost touch. We had fallen off our respective Christmas card "A" lists, replaced by co-workers, bosses, and in-laws.

But everyone has a "B" list, a wish list, comprised of the names of people who really matter in life—names you wish you could keep in your life if only you had. . . .

"The time!" I gasped, looking at my watch. "Look, I've really got to go. I promised my boy I'd . . . "

"No problem," he said. "I understand. I'll be seeing you at class next week anyway."

"Until next week, then. See ya."

On the way home I realized how exhilarated I was at seeing my old friend, and that I didn't want him to remain on my life's "B" list.

I was able, with the help of my course instructor, to learn where he could be found. I looked him up the next day.

"It's good to see you," he said with surprise as he invited me into his living room. "Please, make yourself comfortable."

I felt kind of uneasy, as I'm sure he did, at this business of reacquainting ourselves. After a brief visit, I asked if I could drop by again soon.

"Anytime," he said, with a sincerity reserved for a true friend.

I took him up on his standing invitation almost daily, and before long I realized how these visits somehow helped my pain. Just like my weekly visits to the pain management class did. Only soon the visits with my classmates would end. I will miss them terribly, but I will continue to see my friend. All I have to do is post the sign:

PLEASE DO NOT DISTURB
I'M RELAXING PER MY DOCTOR'S ORDERS

—Bruce R. Comes

Thief

Alone, reluctant I entered the room
To sit among you
And become a thief.
Surreptitiously I observed your tears, listened to your laughter,
and heard your exclamations of recognition.

Furtively I gathered these riches,
Even as I slyly exchanged a shard of childhood joys,
A fragment of adult knowledge,
And placed your precious metals within a velvet purse
To carry in my exit unrepentant.

Perhaps you will forgive my theft,
Realizing at unresolved, unspecified future times
That I like an ailing, confused alchemist will spread
before me the treasures you presented and
Convert your platinum and gold to resurrected life and
rediscover with each revival what I stole:
The Release, Insights, Understanding, Security, the Comfort
To which
Your tears, your laughter, your exclamations
Have been transformed and stored.

Silently, I leave the room
My velvet purse no longer empty, I no longer reluctant, or alone.

—Richard Cohen

Thanks

Thanks for the wonderful trips to the beach—
It's given my mind some much-needed peace.

Even before this course, you see
I knew I was my worst ENEMY!

Anxiety, pain, depression too—
Similar to what all of you were going through.

I needed help; my patience worn thin,
The workbook showed me where to begin.

The weekly homework I did not shirk,
Mentally it was a lot of work.

How far I've come from that first day—
Looking at life in a whole new way.

Old beliefs discarded, changed attitudes I find
I'm doing my spring cleaning, but this year—of my mind!

So "thank you," my two teachers
And all the rest of you.

And as we leave I hear two voices:
"Remember now, you all have choices."

—Carol Rust

Now it's your turn to write a poem or a short prose piece:

Common Chronic Pain Conditions

Chapter 2 defines chronic pain in very broad terms—basically, as pain that lasts for more than three months. As you have seen, chronic pain has almost universal biopsychosocial consequences, no matter what its causes may be. Thus the development of the pain program presented in this book.

I would like to take this opportunity, however, to comment on some of the most common or perhaps least understood pain syndromes I've seen. Although I respect the power of the skills and attitudes presented in this book, I believe that state-of-the art medical treatment must be included in the treatment of chronic pain. I am also aware that there is considerable misinformation about chronic pain syndromes among health care professionals. Therefore, I have chosen the particular syndromes discussed here for one or more of three reasons:

1. They are frequently overlooked.
2. Certain aspects of their cause or treatment are not well known by health care professionals.
3. There are medical treatments, usually aimed at the abnormality contributing to the pain syndrome, that might help reduce the pain experience.

Fibromyalgia

Fibromyalgia is a chronic pain syndrome that affects primarily women (the ratio of women to men with fibromyalgia is 10 to 1). Many terms are used to describe this syndrome, and overlaps among several of the terms suggest points along a symptom continuum. These terms include "fibrositis," "myofascial pain," "postviral fatigue syndrome," "chronic fatigue syndrome," "tension myalgia," and "generalized tendomyopathy." In 1990, the American College of Rheumatology (see Wolfe et al., in Appendix B) developed the following criteria for the classification of fibromyalgia:

1. History of widespread pain.
2. Pain in 11 of 18 tender point sites on digital palpation.

For classification purposes, patients are said to have fibromyalgia if both criteria are satisfied. Widespread pain must have been present for at least three months. The presence of a second clinical disorder does not exclude the diagnosis of fibromyalgia, but the diagnosis is made many times after other diseases have been excluded (e.g., thyroid disease, lupus, rheumatoid arthritis, etc.).

Many patients with fibromyalgia will also have associated complaints, such as sleep disturbance, headache, irritable bowel, irritable bladder, painful menstrual periods, intermittent blurred vision, and short-term memory problems. These complaints imply that the disorder involves more than the musculoskeletal system.

The symptoms are quite variable and are marked by their intermittent, waxing–waning, and migratory pattern. This probably contributes to the long lag time between development of symptoms and diagnosis. The cause is unknown but may be related to changes in the way sensory signals in the spinal cord or brain are processed as the result of neuroplasticity (the ability of the nervous system to alter its connections in response to certain stimuli). The other possibility is that it is the result of interactions between the brain, spinal cord, and immune system that have gone awry. The two most consistent complaints besides pain are sleep disturbance and depression. Therapies directed at these two complaints can be helpful but not curative.

The treatment to date has focused on the sleep disorder by using drugs such as imipramine, amitriptyline, nortriptyline, or cyclobenzaprine to make Stage IV sleep, or restorative sleep, better. Some patients have found SAMe (S-adenosylmethionine), a biological agent with anti-inflammatory and antidepressant properties, helpful. Regular, moderate exercise, such as warm-water pool aerobics, can be very beneficial. In our experience and that of others, the use of cognitive-behavioral therapies such as those presented in this book are associated with improvements in pain, fibromyalgia-related symptoms, and functioning, and with lessening of depression.

Many communities have support groups for fibromyalgia, and your state's Arthritis Foundation may sponsor such groups in your locale. The Arthritis Foundation also sponsors warm-water pool aerobics nationally. Information about these activities, as well as about fibromyalgia syndrome, can be obtained through your state chapter of the Arthritis Foundation. There is also an informative, proactive newsletter available from the Fibromyalgia Network, which makes a good effort to report the latest developments and advocates for more research funding. For more information on how to subscribe to this newsletter, write to the Fibromyalgia Network, P.O. Box 31750, Tucson, AZ 85751-1750; or call (800) 853-2929, fax (520) 290-5550, http://www.fmnetnews.com.

Chronic Neck and Low Back Pain

The causes of chronic pain in the neck or low back can be very challenging to treat. This is particularly so if no structural abnormalities are found, such as a herniated disc, a tumor (a common fear of many who have developed chronic pain syndromes), or significant bony abnormalities of the spine (arthritis with or without clear nerve pinching or fractures). Many times repeated low-back surgeries performed for complaints of continued pain do not result in pain relief. This fact has caused many surgeons to recommend conservative or nonsurgical treatment if only pain is present. If no nervous system abnormalities are present in addition to the pain or if there is no evidence that a deteriorated disc is the source of pain, then repeating surgery may not be an option. As techniques improve for assessing dynamic (in motion) structural spine abnormalities and for distinguishing the origins of pain from the multiple structures of the spine (i.e., facets, discs, nerve roots, ligaments, and muscles), more effective treatments should be forthcoming. Preventing disability from neck or back pain demands addressing mind and body processes.

Because I see either the people who have had unsuccessful surgery or those who have "no abnormalities" on X-ray or MRI studies, I have developed a different way of looking at these individuals in an attempt to discover whether there is some other treatable reason for their symptoms.

In postsurgical patients whose pain is not coming from scar tissue pressing on a nerve or from an unstable spine, and in those patients without any surgically correctable problem, the pain is contributed to by deconditioning of both the abdominal and back muscles. In addition, poor body mechanics and misalignment may contribute to abnormal forces on sensitized nerves and soft tissue. A good conditioning program to strengthen the muscles of the abdomen and back can be very beneficial. For alignment problems and poor body mechanics, treatment with a manual physical therapist who is familiar with such techniques as myofascial release, Jones trigger point therapy, and muscle energy techniques can be very helpful. The use of Alexander and Feldenkrais therapies can be useful for poor body mechanics as well.

One of my frustrations as a pain specialist has been the realization that physical therapists and physical therapy treatments vary enormously. Physical therapy, like many medical disciplines, is very much an art. I recommend asking for a physical therapist who is familiar with treating chronic pain. This means identifying a physical therapist who is comfortable with the possibility of not providing total pain relief—one who can teach you about your body mechanics and how your body moves and who is aware of the importance of developing a long-term maintenance program that you will be able to do indefinitely. I do not expect the therapist to persist in treatment once you have stopped responding or progressing or if you do not do your home program.

Chiropractic treatment in chronic neck and back pain is controversial in terms of its long-term benefits. Evidence has been presented that in acute flare-ups of low back pain this form of treatment can be quite beneficial for some individuals. I believe that chiropractic and manipulative medicine has been instrumental in stimulating the dialogue that is now taking place on the contribution of abnormal body mechanics to neck and back pain, particularly in those acute and chronic pain patients with no X-ray abnormalities (in the conventional sense).

Many chronic neck pain problems are complicated by what is referred to as soft tissue/myofascial pain. After traumatic events such as motor vehicle accidents and lifting injuries, many of my patients with chronic neck pain report not sleeping well, and they have multiple tender points in the muscles of the neck, on the top of shoulders, the trapezius muscle, and in between the shoulder blades. In addition to physical therapy that addresses posture and conditioning of the upper back and extremities, medication to induce restorative sleep can be helpful (e.g., amitriptyline, desipramine). Limited trigger point injections with an anesthetic and/or steroids may be of benefit for initial treatment, and if there is evidence of facet arthritis (the little joints that connect each spinal vertebrae together), facet injections may also be of help.

Headaches

Hundreds of books and research papers have been written, and many clinics have been created, to help with the very common and disabling problem of headaches. Fortunately, most headache syndromes are chronic but intermittent problems. As in the case of back pain, multiple factors are possible as triggers or causes. Over the past decade there have been considerable advances in the understanding of headache causes. The old distinction between migraines and tension-type headaches as vascular and muscular, respectively, is gone. It is believed that most primary headache disorders, such as migraines, cluster headaches, and daily tension-type headaches, come from disturbances in the central nervous system and represent different presentations along a continuum. Because of this complexity, I would strongly recommend, if you are experiencing chronic daily headaches or difficult-to-control, intermittent migraine headaches, that you seek assistance from a headache specialist, usually a neurologist with an interest and expertise in headache management.

There are several behavioral considerations, however, that can be mentioned here that may help you now or prepare you for your specialist visit. Keeping a headache diary of frequency and quality, like the general pain diary, will assist you in recognizing patterns and associations with triggers. Most effective headache treatments are categorized into prophylaxis (prevention), mild to moderate headache treatment, and severe headache treatment. Be aware that the overconsumption of caffeine and the chronic daily use of acetominophen, Fiorecet®, Fiorinol®, and Esgic® or pain medications may lead to "rebound headaches" (i.e., headaches associated with the chronic use of these substances or medications). In addition, Fiorecet®, Fiorinol®, and Esgic® contain barbiturate-like components that may be habit forming and may cause seizures upon sudden cessation of the medication if daily doses are significant. Therefore, slowly decreasing daily doses of such medication is important and should be done with the assistance of your health care professional. Use of these medications or substances should be limited to two to three days per week.

The avoidance of long fasting periods during the day can be helpful to those individuals who may be prone to low blood sugar. Skipping meals is often associated with headaches in susceptible individuals. Finally, constipation may also be associated with chronic daily headaches. Increasing fluids, dietary fiber, exercise, and judicious use of stool softeners may be helpful. More aggressive bowel regimens may be necessary for those using opioids (narcotics). Ask your health care professional for assistance.

When I see patients with complaints of daily headaches, I frequently find that they are suffering from muscle tension or spasm of their neck muscles. Variations on this theme are patients with temporomandibular joint strain caused by clenching or grinding of their teeth; a night guard for the teeth may be helpful in such a case. Therapy directed at strengthening of the upper extremities and good posturing of the head, neck, and upper back are extremely valuable, sometimes eliminating the problem altogether. Patients who experience increased headaches after exercising their upper extremities should take special care, as they are probably using muscles incorrectly because of weakness and straining, and they should have supervision at the beginning.

Interstitial Cystitis

Interstitial cystitis is a disease of the bladder associated with stretch-induced hemorrhaging of the bladder wall that may be associated with frequency of urination (both day and night), pelvic pain, and burning on urination. The condition is seen primarily in women, and the cause is unknown, although recent research has implicated the presence of substance P to be a factor. Substance P is a normal pain-producing chemical commonly seen in inflammatory responses. The urine is negative for infection, although the symptoms of a chronic urinary tract infection are reported, and women may be treated for months to years before interstitial cystitis is discovered. The diagnosis is usually made by passing a scope into the bladder (cystoscopy), looking at the bladder wall for microhemorrhages, and taking a sample of tissue (biopsy). Treatment is available but does not always resolve or help the symptoms. There are national and local organizations to support individuals with interstitial cystitis and to keep them informed as to the latest research and treatment developments. I strongly recommend identifying a urologist who is familiar and comfortable with treating interstitial cystitis. Contact the Interstitial Cystitis Association, 51 Monroe St., Suite 1402, Rockville, MD 20850; or call (301) 610-5300, fax (301) 610-5308, http://www.ichelp.org, for names of health care professionals closest to you or for more information.

Endometriosis

Endometriosis is present in 15–40% of women undergoing laparoscopy for pelvic pain. There is no correlation between location of disease, site or amount of disease, and the presence of pain. Endometriosis is a disorder of women involving the appearance of uterine tissue (endometrium) outside of the uterine cavity (womb). It is unknown why the tissue becomes embedded in areas outside of the uterus. The pain associated with endometriosis is thought to be the result of the microhemorrhages that occur with the monthly menstrual cycle and the resultant irritation of surrounding tissue. However, because the number of abnormal tissue implants does not correlate with the amount, intensity, or frequency of the pelvic pain experienced, there are most likely several mechanisms for pain production (i.e., immune complexes or internal organ sensitization of pain pathways similar to that occurring in neuropathy). Treatments may vary from simple birth control pills to testosterone-like medications to hysterectomy with removal of ovaries. Such hormonal manipulations may be quite successful. There are cases, however, in which endometrial lesions may persist in spite of removal of the ovaries and in which pain persists after removal of the uterus and ovaries. In addition, except for extensive adhesions (internal scar tissue) or those adhesions associated with bowel obstruction, repeated surgeries for cutting and removing those adhesions rarely gives long-term relief. For chronic pelvic pain associated with the presence of endometriosis, therapy should address body, mind, and spirit. This pain syndrome also has national and local groups for patient support and information resources. Contact the Endometriosis Association at 8585 North 76th Place, Milwaukee, WI 53223, http://www.endometriosisassn.org, or call (414) 355-2200 for more information.

Neuropathies

Postherpetic Neuralgia

Several well-known pain conditions are associated with nerve damage or irritation and are thus known as "neuropathies." One of these is postherpetic neuralgia. This is caused by the same virus that causes chicken pox, herpes zoster. It can infect any peripheral nerve and is associated with a funny sensation of the skin, followed by a small blistery rash that over the course of about two weeks becomes crusted and weepy. It may be associated with fever and flu-like symptoms. In individuals over 65 years of age, there is a high likelihood of developing nerve pain that lasts long after the rash has gone. Currently, it is recommended that older individuals at high risk receive nerve blocks from an anesthetist within days to weeks after the rash appears. Another potentially effective treatment is to apply Zostrix® to the painful skin five times a day after the rash has healed. Follow the instructions in the box. Zostrix® is available without a prescription, but consult your health care provider to confirm the diagnosis. For individuals who have developed chronic pain from shingles (postherpetic neuralgia), application of the 5% Lidoderm® patch to involved skin may be symptomatically beneficial. The patch is applied for 12 hours at a time and then removed for 12 hours.

Painful Diabetic Neuropathy

Diabetes can be associated with a painful neuropathy, in addition to the neuropathy characterized by numbness in the hands and lower extremities. Most of the painful diabetic neuropathies are time-limited and "burn out" after 12 to 18 months. Amitriptyline, baclofen, and mexiletine are medications used for this condition that may help.

Complex Regional Pain Syndrome (CRPS), Type I

Sympathetically mediated pain, also known as "reflex sympathetic dystrophy," "Sudeck's dystrophy," or "hand/shoulder syndrome," and now CRPS, Type I, is a condition that can develop after major or minor trauma to the extremities. It is unclear what the true abnormality is, but the result is that the sympathetic nervous system—which controls blood vessel diameter and leakiness, as well as sweating in the extremities—becomes involved in the pain process as well. Thus the syndrome is characterized by swelling, increased sweating, blood vessel constriction (causing the skin to turn dark red to blue), or dilation (causing the skin to turn red and hot and to burn), and severe pain in the involved extremity. Even light touch can cause excruciating pain. It is a very complicated syndrome and needs to be treated by pain specialists or by someone familiar with the diagnosis. I mention it so that if you have such symptoms but have not been diagnosed as yet, you can bring this description to the attention of your health care professional. Sometimes nerve blocks aimed at blocking the sympathetic nervous system can be very effective in altering this pain syndrome, but early intervention appears to be critical. Medications used to help treat symptoms related to this condition are blood pressure pills (such as calcium channel blockers or alpha-adrenergic blockers), antiseizure medications (such as gabapentin or Topamax®), and tricyclic antidepressants (such as amitriptyline or desipramine). Physical therapy, use of contrast baths, desensitization of the painful limb are very important so that function can be maintained. A high-voltage galvanic skin stimulator, may also help with pain and swelling.

Complementary Alternative Medicine

The term "complementary alternative medicine" (CAM) has been used to mean anything outside of the traditionally Western high-tech, pharmaceutical medical system. As a result there has been considerable confusion about what works and how and when to use such therapies. This entire workbook could be called an "alternative, complementary" approach to pain management because it is based on many of the therapies considered to be CAM therapies, such as mind–body therapy, relaxation techniques, and self-help therapies. The power of such therapies is the healing that they can promote: healing in the sense of finding comfort, joy, and purpose in living with a problem such as chronic pain.

There are additional CAM therapies that are similar to our interventions, such as acupuncture and drug treatments in the form of biological agents and herbs. These additional therapies can reduce symptoms, though they do not cure the underlying disease.

Acupuncture

Traditional acupuncture involves the insertion of slender needles into specific points on the body. The needles may be heated with an herb (a process called moxibustion) or electrified. The rationale for point selection is based on numerous interpretations, and you may find an acupuncturist who describes his or her therapy in terms of nationality (e.g., Chinese, Japanese, French, or Korean) or energy system (five elements, Qi [chi]). Many people find that acupuncture is able to reduce tension and pain flare-ups and to increase energy. There has been some research that indicates that acupuncture can safely reduce neck pain and pain in the knees from osteoarthritis. More research studies are actively being performed to further clarify what works.

Treatment by a licensed or certified acupuncturist may assist you with symptom control. Many acupuncturists use disposable needles to reduce risk of infection. In general, some improvement in symptoms would be expected after 8 to 12 treatment sessions.

Biological Agents

Biological agents are those that are actually already synthesized in the body. The ones discussed here are glucosamine, chondroitin 4-sulfate, and SAMe. To date none of the biological agents that have been promoted for treatment of pain have been approved by the Food and Drug Administration (FDA), meaning that safety and effectiveness have not been standardized before their release to the public. As a result a major problem is that preparations vary widely in the amount of active ingredient they contain, and long-term side effects (in years) are unknown (though Europeans have been using such remedies for years).

Glucosamine

Glucosamine sulfate is derived from chitin (the shells of shrimp, lobster, or crab) or synthesized. Evidence exists that glucosamine sulfate can decrease osteoarthritis pain and may stimulate cartilage production. The most frequently used oral dosage is 500 mg three times a day for at least two months. Side effects are rare and usually involve nausea or indigestion.

Chondroitin 4-Sulfate

Chondroitin 4-sulfate is a glycosaminoglycan and is a component of cartilage. Supplements are derived from the cartilage of cattle or sharks. Evidence exists that chondroitin 4-sulfate taken at doses of 400 mg three times a day for two to three months can decrease pain in osteoarthritis. It may also slow cartilage breakdown. Side effects are rare and usually involve nausea or indigestion. It is structurally similar to blood thinners, and caution may be needed with individuals who are taking prescribed blood thinners. Many supplement preparations that contain both glucosamine and chondroitin 4-sulfate are sold. To date there is no evidence that the combined preparation gives additional benefit.

SAMe

SAMe, or S-adenosylmethionine, is a naturally occurring compound synthesized from amino acid L-methionine and adenosine triphosphate (ATP). It plays a role in various metabolic processes and is thought to be possibly both anti-inflammatory and cartilage protective. It has also been thought to have a mild antidepressant effect. Several randomized controlled research trials have demonstrated pain reductions equivalent to those of anti-inflammatory drugs for up to two years with continued benefit in patients with osteoarthritis.

Herbal Remedies

Because of their widespread availability, millions of people have embraced self-medication with herbs in multiple preparations, from teas to capsules. Although most preparations are probably safe, some herbal compounds, such as those containing ephedra, an adrenalin-like substance, have been associated with illness and death. The active therapeutic ingredients in herbal preparations are like drugs. Many of our current medications had their origin in compounds isolated from plants (e.g., digitalis from the foxglove plant, salicylic acid [or aspirin] from willow bark).

Some of the more popular herbs used by patients in chronic pain have been St. John's wort (for mild depression), valerian and kava kava (for sleep), cayenne pepper (used externally, for anti-inflammatory effect), ginger (for inflammation and pain relief), and feverfew for migraines. Several resources can be used to explore the recommended use and effects of a variety of herbal substances; they are included in "Supplementary Reading." The Arthritis Foundation has very good advice about herbs and other CAM therapies in The Arthritis Foundation's Guide to Alternative Therapies. Current research into herbal preparations used in Chinese and Ayurvedic (from India) medicine may shed light on the active ingredient(s) that make them helpful in the treatment of a variety of symptoms.

Massage

Many techniques fall into the category of massage therapy—for example, Swedish, acupressure, lymphatic, reflexology. These techniques apply pressure using the hands to areas of the body to release tension in muscles or prescribed points that are representative of body parts (foot/hand reflexology) or acupuncture points (Shiatsu, Do'in, acupressure). Many people with or without chronic pain find that massage can be helpful to release tension, treat flare-ups, or just relax. Some patients with fibromyalgia may find that they can tolerate only light touch, so it may be important to find a therapist with experience in treating patients with chronic pain and to use your communication skills for treatment feedback.

Energy Therapies

Therapeutic touch, reiki, qi gong and polarity therapy are all techniques that describe their treatment in terms of working with an individual's energy. Although there has been no evidence that these therapies do more than assist the individual in deep relaxation, many patients find the treatment comforting and helpful in relieving fatigue and tension. Many of the practitioners of these therapies also help the individuals being treated to reproduce the healing effects on their own, which can add to an individual's resources of pain coping skills.

Supplementary Reading

Judith Horstman, *The Arthritis Foundation's Guide to Alternative Therapies* (Atlanta, GA: Arthritis Foundation, 1999).

David Sobel and Robert Ornstein, *The Healthy Mind Healthy Body Handbook* (Los Altos, CA: Malor Books, 1997).

Andrew Weil, *Health and Healing: Understanding Conventional and Alternative Medicine* (Boston: Houghton Mifflin, 1998).

Publications from the National Center for Complementary and Alternative Medicine:
NCCAM Clearinghouse
P.O. Box 8218
Silver Spring, MD 20907-8218
1-888-644-6226
http://nccam.nih.gov/

Working Comfortably

Nancy L. Josephson

Many patients who participate in the pain program work in offices and use computers on a daily basis. If you are one of these patients, correctly setting up your computer work area so that you are comfortable is very important in reducing or preventing the following:

- Neck and shoulder pain
- Eyestrain
- Stiffness
- Carpal tunnel syndrome
- Wrist pain
- Back pain
- Headaches
- Repetitive strain injury

Most larger companies are very "ergonomically aware" of correctly setting up work areas. If you are fortunate enough to work for such a company, take advantage of the services it offers. Even if your company does not offer ergonomic services, you can set up your own office so it is comfortable for you to work in.

Adjusting Your Chair

The best type of chair for office work is a "secretarial" chair (no arms) that has four types of adjustments:

- Seat height
- Seat angle
- Back height
- Back angle

Use the following guidelines when adjusting your chair:

1. Adjust the seat height so that your knees are bent at an angle of slightly over 90° and your feet are comfortable flat on the floor.
2. Don't cross your legs while working. That can constrict blood flow, causing tingling and making your legs "go to sleep."
3. Adjust the seat angle of your chair so that there is not a great deal of pressure on the part of your upper leg just above the knee.
4. Try to avoid chairs with arms. They put extra pressure on your arms and also position them at an unnatural angle if you tend to rest your arms on them.
5. You may need further lower back support than your chair provides. Check with your physician or physical therapist for recommendations of back support pillows that best suit your needs.

Adjusting the Monitor Height and Distance

Now that your chair is comfortable, move it to your desk and sit down. You're now going to adjust the height of your monitor so less stress is placed on your neck and shoulders.

1. Sit comfortably on your chair. Keep your feet flat on the floor.
2. Hold your head so that you are looking straight ahead, not down and not up. This is the position your head should maintain when looking at the monitor. Relax your shoulders and arms while you are doing this.
3. Raise or lower the height of your monitor so that you are looking straight ahead—neither up nor down. The monitor height should be approximately the same as your forehead height. You can raise the height of your monitor in a variety of ways:

   - Telephone books
   - Packages of paper
   - Catalogues
   - Specially designed shelving

4. The viewing distance from your eyes to the monitor should be 16–24 inches.

5. If the angle of your monitor can be adjusted, try tilting it 10–20°.

6. Once you have set the height of your monitor, sit down and see whether the position is comfortable for you. If you feel stress on your neck, try raising or lowering the monitor until it is comfortable for you.

Preventing Glare

Glare is the biggest single cause of eyestrain when a computer is being used. It is relatively easy to avoid eyestrain by following these suggestions:

1. Avoid setting your monitor in direct light (sunlight, overhead light, etc.).

2. Fluorescent overhead lights are the biggest culprits in causing glare. If possible, have the ones directly over your monitor turned off. You can always use a small portable light for desktop lighting if necessary.

3. Various types of glare screens are available at your local computer store. These can easily be attached directly to the front of your monitor.

4. Eyeglasses for glare prevention are also available, even for people who do not wear prescription glasses. Check with your ophthalmologist for suggestions.

5. Something as simple as a large piece of cardboard that extends over the top of your monitor can help reduce glare.

6. Avoid staring at the screen for too long a period of time. People who do this tend not to blink as often; this causes dry, hot eyes. Look away and focus on an object at a distance for a few seconds. Blink frequently to avoid dryness.

Adjusting the Keyboard Height

Carpal tunnel syndrome and repetitive strain injury have become the fashionable ailments of the 1990s, thanks to keyboards and mouse devices. If you use a keyboard or mouse device, you are susceptible to these problems, but your chances of getting them can be greatly reduced by a proper keyboard height. Follow these guidelines when setting up your keyboard:

1. The table height of your work surface should be between 23 and 28 inches (floor to typing surface).

2. Use a comfortable wrist pad in front of your keyboard, so that your wrists lie comfortably on the pad instead of the hard tabletop.

3. Adjust the table height so that when you position your hands on the keyboard, your elbows are bent at a 90° angle and your wrists are not bent up or down. Make sure that your wrists lie flat and that your fingers are stretched out in front.

Using a Mouse Pad

If you use a mouse device, follow these suggestions to prevent wrist and shoulder stress:

1. Use a mouse pad to protect your mouse and make it easier for you to operate the mouse.
2. Try to move your entire arm when using a mouse. Many people make sharp, jerky movements with just their wrists when using a mouse. This puts added stress on the wrist.
3. Take a "mouse break" every now and then.
4. Position the mouse pad next to the keyboard so you don't have to reach too far for the mouse.

Taking Breaks

If you spend more than an hour a day at your computer, the best thing you can do for your body and mind is to take breaks. Most computers have built-in clocks, and you can set an alarm that will tell you it's time to take a break. Determine how long you can work comfortably before you need to take a break. Then take that break!

Exercising

Exercising is also a good way to reduce stress while you are working at a computer. Here are a few exercises that you can try:

Breathing

Perform diaphragmatic breathing to help relax your body and to reduce stress and tension. Let your head relax along with your shoulders and arms.

Eye Exercises

1. Look away from your monitor and focus on an object at a distance for a few seconds.
2. Blink your eyes frequently to provide moisture.
3. Move your eyes to the left, then to the right. Look up and then down.

Stretching Exercises

The following exercises can help reduce any tension or muscle strain that occurs while using your computer.

Shoulders and Neck

1. Raise your shoulders toward your ears, and hold that slight tension for just a moment.
2. Relax your shoulders and arms.
3. Repeat this five times to prevent tightness in the shoulder and neck area.

Upper Back

1. Make sure you are sitting up straight.
2. Put your hands behind your head so that your elbows point out to the side.
3. Pull your shoulder blades toward each other until you feel a slight tightness in your upper back.
4. Hold this for about 10 seconds. Then release and relax.

Hands

There are two exercises for the hands. Here is the first:

1. Make a tight fist.
2. Hold for a few seconds.
3. Relax your hands.

And the second:

1. Straighten your fingers out in front of you.
2. Spread them as far apart from one another as you can.
3. Hold the spread until you feel slight tension.
4. Relax.

General Stretching

A good general exercise is just to get up from your desk and walk around, swinging your arms and moving your body.

Appendix D

Bibliography

This appendix contains a complete list of all the books and articles recommended in the "Supplementary Reading" sections of various chapters, plus some additional resources.

Aaron Antonovsky, *Unraveling the Mystery of Health: How People Manage Stress and Stay Well* (San Francisco: Jossey-Bass,1987). Out of print.

American Heart Association, *American Heart Association Low-Fat, Low Cholesterol Cookbook: Heart Healthy, Easy to Make Recipes That Taste Great* (New York: Times Books, 1998).

Americans with Disabilities Act Handbook [Resources for employment] (Equal Employment Opportunity Commission and Justice Department 1992). Available at bookstores, disAbility.gov, or http://disability.gov/CSS/Default.asp.

Paul Arnstein, Margaret Caudill, Carol Lynn Mandle, A. Norris, and Ralph Beasley, "Self-Efficacy as a Mediator of the Relationship Between Pain Intensity, Disability and Depression in Chronic Pain Patients," *Pain,* 81: 483–491, 1999.

Lorna Bell and Eudora Seyfer, *Gentle Yoga* (Berkeley, CA: Celestial Arts, 1987).

Herbert Benson, *The Relaxation Response* (New York: Mass Market Paperback, 1990).

Herbert Benson and Eileen Stuart, *The Wellness Book: The Comprehensive Guide to Maintaining Health and Treating Stress-Related Illness* (New York: Fireside, 1993).

Niels Becker, Per Sjogren, Per Bech, Alf Kornelius Olsen and Jorgen Eriksen, "Treatment Outcome of Chronic Non-malignant Pain Patients Managed in a Danish Multidisciplinary Pain Centre Compared to General Practice: A Randomised Controlled Trial," *Pain,* 84: 203–211, 2000.

Nicola Biller, Paul Arnstein, Margaret Caudill, Carol Wells-Federman, and Carolyn Guberman, "Predicting Completion of a Cognitive-Behavioral Pain Management Program by Initial Measures of a Chronic Pain Patient's Readiness for Change," *Clinical Journal of Pain*, *16*(4): 352–359, 2000.

Joan Borysenko, *Minding the Body, Mending the Mind* (New York: Bantam Doubleday Dell Publications, 1993).

David Burns, *The Feeling Good Handbook* (New York: Plume, 1999).

David Burns, *Ten Days to Self-Esteem* (New York: Quill/William Morrow, 1999).

Margaret Caudill, Richard Schnable, Patricia Zuttermeister, Herbert Benson, and Richard Friedman, "Decreased Clinic Use by Chronic Pain Patients: Response to Behavioral Medicine Interventions," *Clinical Journal of Pain*, *7*: 305–310, 1991.

Robert Cialdini, *Influence: The Psychology of Persuasion* (New York: Quill/William Morrow, 1993).

L. Gail Darlington, "Dietary Therapy for Arthritis," *Rheumatic Disease Clinics of North America*, *17*: 273–285, 1991.

Gail Darlington and Linda Gamlin, *Diet and Arthritis* (N. Pomfret, VT: Trafalgar Square, 1998).

Martha Davis, Elizabeth Robbins Eshelman, and Matthew McKay, *The Relaxation and Stress Reduction Workbook* (Oakland, CA: New Harbinger Publications, 2000).

Thomas Delbanco, "Enriching the Doctor–Patient Relationship by Inviting the Patient's Perspective," *Annals of Internal Medicine, 116*: 414–418, 1992.

Johanna Dwyer, "Nutritional Remedies: Reasonable and Questionable," *Annals of Behavioral Medicine, 14*: 120–125, 1992.

L. D. Egbert, G. E. Battit, C. E. Welch, and M. K. Bartlett, "Reduction in Post-operative Pain by Encouragement and Instruction of Patients: A Study of Doctor–Patient Rapport," *New England Journal of Medicine, 270*: 825–827, 1964.

Paul Ekman, Robert Levenson, and Wallace Friesen, "Autonomic Nervous System Activity Distinguishes among Emotions," *Science, 221*: 1208–1210, 1983.

Albert Ellis, *How to Make Yourself Happy and Remarkably Less Disturbable* (Manassas Park, VA: Impact Publications, 1999).

Patrick Fanning, *Visualization for Change* (Oakland, CA: New Harbinger Publications, 1994).

Fawzy I. Fawzy, Nancy Fawzy, Christine Hyun, Robert Elashoff, Donald Guthrie, John Fahey, and Donald Morton, "Malignant Melanoma: Effects of an Early Structured Psychiatric Intervention, Coping, and Affective State on Recurrence and Survival 6 Years Later," *Archives of General Psychiatry, 50*: 681–688, 1993.

Howard L. Fields, *Pain Mechanisms and Management, Second Edition* (New York: McGraw-Hill, 2001).

Roger Fisher and William Ury, *Getting to Yes: Negotiating Agreement without Giving In* (New York: Penguin, 1991).

Beverly Flanigan, *Forgiving the Unforgivable: Overcoming the Bitter Legacy of Intimate Wounds* (New York: Macmillan, 1992).

John Frank, Sandra Sinclair, Shielah Hogg-Johnson, Harry Shannon, Claire Bombadier, Dorcas Beaton, and Donald Cole, "Preventing Disability from Work-Related Low-Back Pain," *Canadian Medical Journal, 158*: 1625–1631, 1998.

Shakti Gawain, *Creative Visualization* (New York: Bantam Books, 1983).

Brent Q. Hafen, Kathryn J. Frandsen, Keith J. Karren, and Keith Hooker, *The Health Effects of Attitudes, Emotions and Relationships* (Provo, UT: EMS, 1992).

Edward T. Hall, *Beyond Culture* (New York: Anchor, 1977).

Thich Nhat Hanh, *The Miracle of Mindfulness: A Manual of Meditation* (Boston: Beacon Press, 1996).

Christopher W. Hoenig, *The Problem Solving Journey: Your Guide to Making Decisions and Getting Results* (Reading, MA: Perseus Books, 2000).

Judith Horstman, *The Arthritis Foundation's Guide to Alternative Therapies* (Atlanta, GA: The Arthritis Foundation, 1999).

Edmund Jacobson, *Progressive Relaxation* (Chicago: University of Chicago Press, 1938). Out of print.

Jon Kabat-Zinn, *Full Catastrophe Living: Using the Wisdom of Your Body and Mind to Face Stress, Pain, and Illness* (New York: Delacorte Press, 1990).

Jens Kjeldsen-Kragh et al., "Controlled Trial of Fasting and One-Year Vegetarian Diet in Rheumatoid Arthritis," *Lancet, 338*: 899–902, 1991.

Allen Klein, *The Healing Power of Humor* (Los Angeles: Tarcher, 1989).

Suzanne Kobasa, "Stressful Life Events, Personality and Health: An Inquiry into Hardiness," *Journal of Personality and Social Psychology, 37*: 1–11, 1979.

J. M. Kremer et al., "Effects of High Dose Fish Oil on Rheumatoid Arthritis after Stopping Nonsteroidal Anti-inflammatory Drugs: Clinical and Immune Correlates," *Arthritis and Rheumatology, 38*: 1107–1114, 1995.

Carol Krucoff, Mitchell Krucoff, and Adam Brill, *Healing Moves: How to Cure, Relieve, and Prevent Common Ailments with Exercise* (New York: Crown Publishers, 2000).

Loretta Laroche, *Life Is Not a Stress Rehearsal: Bringing Yesterday's Sane Wisdom into Today's Insane World* (New York: Broadway Books, 2001).

Richard S. Lazarus and Susan Folkman, *Stress, Appraisal, and Coping* (New York: Springer, 1984).

Kate Lorig, James Fries, and Maureen Gecht, *The Arthritis Helpbook: A Tested Self-Management Program for Coping with Arthritis and Fibromyalgia* (Reading, MA: Perseus Books, 2000).

Matthew McKay and Peter Rogers, *The Anger Control Workbook* (Oakland, CA: New Harbinger Publications, 2000).

M. A. Minor and M. K. Sanford, "Physical Interventions in the Management of Pain in Arthritis," *Arthritis Care and Research, 6*: 197–206, 1993.

James Moore, Kate Lorig, Michael VanKorff, Virginia Gonzalez, and Diane Laurent, *The Back Pain Helpbook* (Reading, MA: Perseus Books, 1999).

David Morris, *The Culture of Pain* (Berkeley: University of California Press, 1991).

National Center for Complementary and Alternative Medicine. NCCAM Clearinghouse, P.O. Box 8218, Silver Spring, MD 20907-8218; or call 888-644-6226; http://nccam.nih.gov/.

Miriam Nelson, Wendy Wray, and Sarah Wernick, *Strong Women Stay Young* (New York: Bantam Doubleday Dell Publications, 2000).

Portia Nelson, *There's a Hole in My Sidewalk* (Hillsboro, OR: Beyond Words, 1994).

D. C. Nordstrom et al., "Alpha Linoleic Acid in the Treatment of Rheumatoid Arthritis: A Double Blind, Placebo Controlled and Randomized Study: Flaxseed vs. Safflower Oil," *Rheumatology International, 14*: 231–234, 1995.

Nutrition Action Health Letter. For subscription information, write to the Center for Science in the Public Interest, 1875 Connecticut Ave. N.W., Suite 300, Washington, DC 20009–5728; or call (202) 332-9110, fax (202) 265–4954, *cspi@cspinet.org*, http://www.cspinet.org.

Judith K. Ockene, "Physician-Delivered Interventions for Smoking Cessation," *Preventive Medicine, 16*: 723–737, 1987.

Robert Ornstein, *Evolution of Consciousness* (New York: Touchstone, 1992).

Robert Ornstein, *The Psychology of Consciousness* (New York: Penguin Books, 1986).

Robert Ornstein and David Sobel, *The Healing Brain* (Los Altos, CA: Malor Books, 1999).

Robert Ornstein and David Sobel, *Healthy Pleasures* (Reading, MA: Perseus Books, 1990).

Richard Panush, "Does Food Cause or Cure Arthritis?" *Rheumatic Disease Clinics of North America, 17*: 259–272, 1991.

James Pennebaker, *Opening Up: The Healing Power of Expressing Emotions* (New York: Guilford Press, 1997).

Jean A. T. Pennington and Helen Nichols Church, *Bowes and Church's Food Values of Portions Commonly Used,* 13th Edition (New York: Harper & Row, 1980).

Reynolds Price, *A Whole New Life* (New York: Scribner, 2000).

Cynthia Radnitz, "Food Triggered Migraine: A Critical Review," *Annals of Behavioral Medicine, 12*: 51–64, 1990.

James Rainville, David Ahern, Linda Phalen, Lisa Childs, and Robin Sutherland, "The Association of Pain with Physical Activities in Chronic Low Back Pain," *Spine, 17*: 1060–1064, 1992.

James M. Rippe and Ann Ward, *Rockport's Complete Book of Fitness Walking* (New York: Prentice-Hall Press, 1989).

Carl Rogers, *Client-Centered Therapy: Its Current Practice, Implications, and Theory* (Boston: Houghton Mifflin, 1951). Out of print.

Anne Wilson Schaef, *Meditations for Women Who Do Too Much* (San Francisco: Harper, 1996).

Martin Seligman, *Learned Optimism* (New York: Pocket Books, 1998).

Idries Shah, *The Pleasantries of the Incredible Mulla Nasrudin* (London: Octagon Press, 1983).

Idries Shah, *Reflections* (London: Octagon Press, 1983).

Idries Shah, *The Subtleties of the Inimitable Mulla Nasrudin* and *The Exploits of the Incomparable Mulla Nasrudin* (London: Octagon Press, 1989).

David Sobel and Robert Ornstein, *The Healthy Mind Healthy Body Handbook* (Los Altos, CA: Malor Books, 1997).

Jenny Steinmetz, Jon Blankenship, Linda Brown, Deborah Hall, and Grace Miller, *Managing Stress Before It Manages You* (Palo Alto, CA: Bull, 1980).

Deborah Tannen, *That's Not What I Meant! How Conversational Style Makes or Breaks Relationships* (New York: Ballantine Books, 1991).

Deborah Tannen, *You Just Don't Understand: Women and Men in Conversation* (New York: Ballantine Books, 1991).

Tufts University Diet and Nutrition Letter. For subscription information, write to P.O. Box 420235, Palm Coast, FL 32142; or call (800) 274–7581.

Tufts University Nutrition Navigator. http://navigator.tufts.edu.

Dennis Turk, Donald Meichenbaum, and Myles Genest, *Pain and Behavioral Medicine: A Cognitive-Behavioral Perspective* (New York: Guilford Press, 1985).

Patrick Wall and Steven Rose (Eds.), *Pain: The Science of Suffering* (New York: Columbia University Press, 2000).

Hope S. Warshaw and George Blackburn, *The Restaurant Companion: A Guide to Healthier Eating Out* (Chicago: Surrey Books, 1995).

Andrew Weil, *Eating Well for Optimum Health: The Essential Guide to Food, Diet, and Nutrition* (New York: Knopf, 2000).

Andrew Weil, *Health and Healing: Understanding Conventional and Alternative Medicine* (Boston: Houghton Mifflin, 1998).

Hendria Weisinger, *Dr. Weisinger's Anger Workout Book* (New York: Quill, 1985).

Redford B. Williams and Virginia Williams, *Anger Kills: Seventeen Strategies for Controlling the Hostility That Can Harm Your Health* (New York: Harper Mass Market Paperback, 1998).

Denise Winn, *The Manipulated Mind: Brainwashing, Conditioning and Manipulation* (Los Altos, CA: Malor Books, 2000).

Frederick Wolfe et al., "The American College of Rheumatology 1990 criteria for the classification of fibromyalgia," *Arthritis and Rheumatism, 33*: 160–172, 1990.

Index

About the Author

Margaret A. Caudill, MD, PhD, is a board-certified internist and a Diplomate of Pain Medicine. She has served as Co-Director of the Arnold Pain Center, Beth Israel Deaconess Medical Center, Boston, MA, and as Co-Director of the Department of Pain Medicine at Dartmouth Hitchcock, Manchester, NH. Formerly Assistant Professor of Anesthesiology and Critical Care Medicine at Harvard Medical School, she is currently Adjunct Associate Professor of Anesthesiology at Dartmouth Medical School. Dr. Caudill has long been interested in assisting the development of self-efficacy in people with chronic illness through the application of mind–body skills. She has researched and written extensively on mind–body medicine and lectured internationally on the importance of the biopsychosocial treatment model of pain. She lives in New England with her husband and two cats and, when not involved in her clinical work, research, and writing, enjoys bird watching, gardening, and cooking with friends.

Worksheets
and Other Materials

Contents

Sample Pain Diary

Name _____

Column headers:
- Describe situation ⟹
- Physical sensation (0–10) ⟹
- Describe physical sensation ⟹
- Emotional response (0–10) ⟹
- Describe emotional response ⟹
- Action taken, including medications ⟹

Monday
Date: 11/1

Time	Describe situation	Physical sensation (0–10)	Describe physical sensation	Emotional response (0–10)	Describe emotional response	Action taken, including medications
Time 1: 8 AM	Breakfast	6	Achey	5	Frustrated	Shower
Time 2: Noon	Lunch	8	Throbbing	8	Disgusted	2 ibuprofen
Time 3: 9 PM	Bedtime	10	Sharp	10	Helpless	Heating pad
Total:		24		23		
Average:		8		8		

Tuesday
Date: 11/2

Time	Describe situation	Physical sensation (0–10)	Describe physical sensation	Emotional response (0–10)	Describe emotional response	Action taken, including medications
Time 1: 8:30 AM	Breakfast	9	Sharp spasms	10	Scared	Go back to bed
Time 2: 11:30 AM	Getting up	7	Throbbing	8	Sad	RR, heat
Time 3: 9 PM	Paying bills	5	Sore	4	Comforted	Paced activities
Total:		21		22		
Average:		7		7		

Wednesday
Date: 11/3

Time	Describe situation	Physical sensation (0–10)	Describe physical sensation	Emotional response (0–10)	Describe emotional response	Action taken, including medications
Time 1: 8 AM	Getting up	4	Sore	2	Relief	Gentle exercise
Time 2: Noon	Lunch	5	Sore	1	In control	RR, 2 aspirin
Time 3: 10 PM	Dinner out	6	Achey	1	Happy	Hot shower on return
Total:		15		4		
Average:		5		1		

Thursday
Date: 11/4

Time	Describe situation	Physical sensation (0–10)	Describe physical sensation	Emotional response (0–10)	Describe emotional response	Action taken, including medications
Time 1: 7:30 AM	Breakfast	5	Achey	1	In control	RR
Time 2: 1 PM	House cleaning	6	Sore	2	In control	Sitting, paying bills
Time 3: 9:30 PM	Watching TV	5	Achey	1	Happy	Stretching
Total:		16		4		
Average:		5		1		

Pain Diary

Name _____

	Describe situation	Physical sensation (0–10)	Describe physical sensation	Emotional response (0–10)	Describe emotional response	Action taken, including medications
Monday Date:						
Time 1:						
Time 2:						
Time 3:						
	Total: Average:		Total: Average:			
Tuesday Date:						
Time 1:						
Time 2:						
Time 3:						
	Total: Average:		Total: Average:			
Wednesday Date:						
Time 1:						
Time 2:						
Time 3:						
	Total: Average:		Total: Average:			

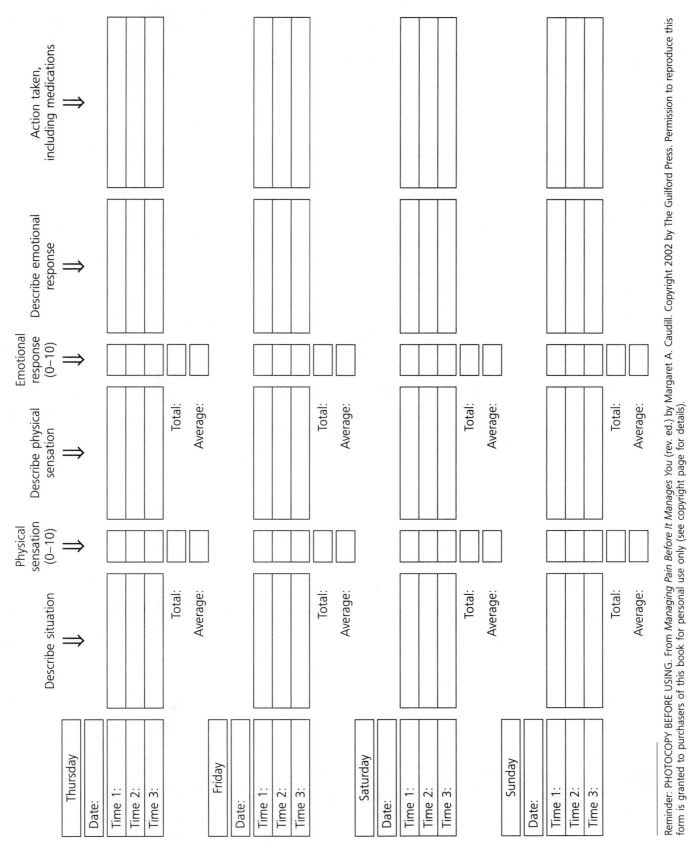

Action taken, including medications ⇒

Describe emotional response ⇒

Emotional response (0–10) ⇒

Describe physical sensation ⇒

Physical sensation (0–10) ⇒

Describe situation ⇒

Thursday

Date:

Time 1:
Time 2:
Time 3:

Total:
Average:

Friday

Date:

Time 1:
Time 2:
Time 3:

Total:
Average:

Saturday

Date:

Time 1:
Time 2:
Time 3:

Total:
Average:

Sunday

Date:

Time 1:
Time 2:
Time 3:

Total:
Average:

Relaxation Response Technique Diary

Complete the following weekly RR Diary. Next to each category indicate the appropriate information about your daily practice. Use this diary for the first three weeks to reinforce practice.

Date							
Time started							
Time stopped							
Place							
Position (e.g., lying down, sitting)							
Degree of relaxation at end (0–10) 0 = very relaxed 10 = very tense							
Effects on pain? Decrease = D Increase = I No change = NC							
Method (tape, exercise, visualization, other)							

Were there any problems that prevented you from practicing the RR daily? How can you solve the problem(s)? _____

_____

_____

_____

_____

_____

_____

_____

_____

Increasing Activities Worksheet

Date: _____ Name: _____

Make a list of activities that increase your pain and those that decrease your pain (refer to Chapter 4).

Activities that increase my pain	**Activities that decrease my pain**
Example: Washing dishes (standing)	Paying bills (sitting)

_____   _____
_____   _____
_____   _____
_____   _____

Can you *delegate* any of the activities associated with pain increases? (For example, bringing dirty laundry to the washing machine.) Star (*) the ones you can.

Delegate one activity this week. It will be _____

Choose one "increase pain" activity and time how long it takes to increase pain level by 2 points. Then choose a "decrease pain" activity from your list and time how long it takes for the pain to decrease again. Alternate between activities that increase and decrease your pain.

Example: Pain ↑ Activity = Wash dishes   Pain ↓ Activity = Pay bills

Wash dishes (10 mins.)   Sort bills from mail (15 mins.)
Wash dishes (10 mins.)   Write checks (15 mins.)
Wash dishes (10 mins.)   Address envelopes (10 mins.)

Activity that increases pain	**Activity that decreases pain**

_____   _____
_____   _____
_____   _____
_____   _____

Can you *adapt* any of the above activities so that they can be performed more easily? What would be some of the adaptations? (For example: sitting to fold laundry or peel vegetables; lying down to call a friend or listen to a book on tape; opening cabinet door under kitchen sink so that you can rest one foot on the shelf; putting bowls in sink to stir ingredients)

_____
_____
_____
_____
_____

Food Diary Instructions

Time started: The time of day that you begin eating a meal.

Food/beverage: Record everything you eat and drink. Note such things as whether the food or beverage contained a sweetener substitute or whether it was a new product for you. Are you eating five servings of fruits and vegetables and six servings of grain products (including whole grains) per day?

Quantity: The amount that you ate or drank (1 cup, 8 oz. glass) or the plate portion (1/2, 1/4 of the dinner plate).

Time ended: The time at which you ended the meal you were recording. (If a number of your meals last 10 minutes or less, maybe you should consider eating more slowly.)

You may have to keep a food diary for many weeks before you see a relationship between foods and pain patterns.

Food Diary

Date: _____ Name: _____

Time started	Food/beverage	Quantity	Time ended

Daily Record of Automatic Thoughts (Self-Talk)

Date	Situation	Automatic thoughts	Physical response	Emotional response	Cognitive distortion	Changed thought

Weekly Feedback Sheet

Name: _____

Date: _____ Reporting for week of: _____

1. Record the daily averages of your physical sensation and emotional response below:

	Day 1	Day 2	Day 3	Day 4	Day 5	Day 6	Day 7	Weekly average
Physical sensation:	____	____	____	____	____	____	____	____
Emotional response:	____	____	____	____	____	____	____	____

If this is your first session, record your pain level now (on a scale of 0–10): ____

2. Over the past week, has your *physical sensation*:

Improved ____   Stayed the same ____   Become worse ____

Why do you think that your *physical sensation* has improved, stayed the same, or become worse?

_____

_____

Over the past week, has your *emotional response*:

Improved ____   Stayed the same ____   Become worse ____

Why do you think that your *emotional response* has improved, stayed the same, or become worse?

_____

_____

3. List all medication you are taking:

Name of medication	Dosage (mg)	Frequency*
_____	_____	_____
_____	_____	_____
_____	_____	_____
_____	_____	_____
_____	_____	_____
_____	_____	_____
_____	_____	_____

*How many times per day or per week do you take each medication?
If you take opioids, how many pills did you take for this week? ____

4. Did you receive any other pain treatments this week—for example, nerve blocks, physical therapy, acupuncture, etc.? _____

_____

_____

5. How many times this week did you do the following?

Relaxation response techniques _____   Mini-relaxations _____

6. For how long and how often did you do physical exercise this week?

Aerobic _____   Time _____   How often? _____

Stretching _____   Time _____   How often? _____

Strengthening _____   Time _____   How often? _____

7. What goal did you set for the week? _____
Did you accomplish it? (Y/N) _____   If you did not accomplish it, can you come up with a contingency plan that might help you succeed by identifying the obstacle and a solution to the obstacle?

Obstacle	Solution
_____	_____
_____	_____
_____	_____
_____	_____

8. Where did you find your pleasure this week? _____

_____

_____

9. Do you have any questions or problems? _____

_____

_____

10. To health care professionals: Is there any other information you wish to collect? Fill in before copying.

_____

_____

_____

_____

_____

_____

_____

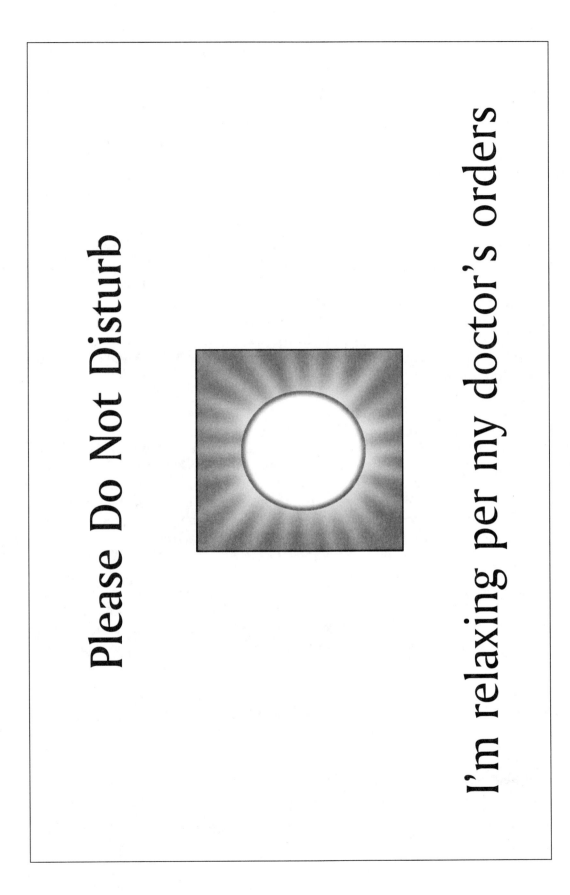

Please Do Not Disturb

I'm relaxing per my doctor's orders

Letter to Health Care Professionals

Dear Health Care Professional:

Managing Pain Before It Manages You is a practical, patient-oriented workbook. It provides information on basic pain mechanisms, medical treatment of chronic pain, and multiple cognitive behavioral skills that can assist coping and functioning. This book can be used by patients alone but can be even more effective if supported by a health care professional who can guide the patient through the program and reinforce the book's information. The workbook was originally written to supplement a 10-visit group medical program for chronic pain management, but it can be used in individual therapy as well.

If you are a physician, nurse practitioner, or physician assistant, this book can supplement the pharmacological, interventional, and surgical treatments recommended to patients with chronic pain.

If you are a psychologist, social worker, or nurse, this workbook offers a complete, self-guided cognitive behavioral therapy program for your clients or patients. It may be used in patient education, in conjunction with other medical therapies, and in psychotherapy. Patients can use the workbook independently or as a formal 8- to 10-week individual or group program.

Efficacy of This Approach

Research has shown that health care professionals can play a critical role in facilitating a patient's response to therapeutic interventions, as well as in changing their behaviors (Egbert et al., 1964; Hafen et al., 1992; Ockene, 1987). For example, encouraging patients to discuss pain from their perspective and giving them information on self-management can increase patient adherence, reduce symptoms, and/or facilitate symptom management (Caudill et al., 1991; Delbanco, 1992). Applying a behavioral medicine model to symptom management acknowledges the complex biology, psychology, and sociology of an illness that needs to be considered in any therapeutic recommendation. The materials presented in this book are grounded in a behavioral medicine model, and they have been demonstrated to decrease symptoms and decrease clinic utilization by patients with chronic pain (Caudill et al., 1991; Becker et al., 2000). Furthermore, this intervention can increase self–efficacy, an important mediator of pain-related disability and depressive symptoms (Arnstein et al., 1999).

The Professional's Role in Facilitating This Program

> Those who do not feel pain, seldom think that it is felt.
> —*Samuel Johnson M.D., 1708–1784*

We can often best help patients with chronic pain by admitting the limits of our knowledge. There is much we don't know about chronic pain mechanisms for prevention or treatment. It is important to believe patients who report their pain experience. There is no objective measure of pain at this time. It is important for you and your patient to acknowledge that although living in pain is a challenge, there are many things that can be done to decrease symptoms and improve quality of life. If you do not feel comfortable evaluating and treating chronic pain, it is your obligation to refer the patient to someone who can.

Assessing and Encouraging Patient Readiness for Change

Teaching an appreciation of the biopsychosocial process from the time of the initial evaluation will lend validity to advising treatment that includes cognitive behavioral therapies. By exploring what other symptoms patients are experiencing in addition to their pain, the professional can help identify other stress-related symptoms, such as fatigue, memory problems, irritable bowel, muscle tension, shortness of breath, palpitations, irritability, and insomnia. Asking other specific questions in the psychosocial history can help get to other influencing issues and provide more mind–body connections for discussion; for example:

- "What functions or activities have been altered by your pain?" Humans are incredibly adaptable and are quite capable of using denial for coping. Detailing work inside and outside the home can give evidence for the magnitude of pain complaints.
- "From whom or what do you get your emotional or problem-solving support?" Behavioral medicine research has documented the positive power of support through close friends, spouses, and religious affiliation. However, many patients with chronic pain suffer isolation and despair.
- "In addition to your pain and dysfunction, what other stresses are you finding yourself having to cope with right now?" This can be a very revealing question. The losses incurred from unemployment or decreased work capacity alone can have economic, social, and self-esteem consequences of enormous importance.
- "Have you ever had a significant incident(s) of physical, emotional, or sexual abuse or trauma?" There is a very high positive response to this question in my practice. Such histories are important to uncover, as they influence how one might approach teaching the relaxation skills and may require individual treatment to put into perspective the differences between feeling vulnerable, not believed, and out of control after having been abused and when in chronic pain.
- "What do you think is going on? Do you have any fears or concerns about your pain?" The majority of patients have ideas (or fears) about the source or cause of their pain. For obvious reasons, addressing them may go along way in obtaining their willingness to see their part in pain management.
- "What do you want to get from your visit with me today?" This can be an important message to the patient that he or she has a right to have expectations regarding a visit and can be a good starting point in clarifying realistic expectations. This can be the perfect opening to discuss the roles of the health care professional and the patient toward reaching a common goal.

- "If I can't cure you today, what would be the next best thing?" This question stems from a common response of many patients to the last question. They will say, "You don't understand, doctor, I don't want my pain, so why would I want to manage it?" This again allows for the discussion of the nature of chronic pain and the reality of persistent pain. Early in treatment many people feel that acceptance of pain management is a condemnation to a life of pain even if a cure comes along, that somehow they will be excluded because they have accepted. This misunderstanding is important to clarify. Acceptance is dealing with the here and now; pain may be mandatory, but the suffering is definitely optional.

These questions can quickly give you an overview of the context of an individual's pain experience and lay the groundwork for establishing that pain is both stressful and affected by stress. It also sends the message that you are concerned about the pain and the person in pain. Listening to the responses of the patient to these questions helps set up realistic treatment expectations and orients treatment to the patient's level of understanding, in the context of his or her pain experience.

Patients in precontemplation (Biller et al., 2000) who have not thought about the relationship between behavior and pain can be asked just to read Chapters 1 through 5 of the workbook, without doing the exercises described. They can also begin keeping a pain diary, as described in Chapter 1, which will help them focus on just how their pain is affected by their daily activities and mood.

Patients are most ready to start *using* this workbook when they can acknowledge: (1) that changing their behavior may help them cope with or manage their pain, or (2) that they need new skills to handle the physical, emotional, and cognitive effects of pain on their lives.

Guiding Patients through the Workbook

When patients are ready for it, this workbook can provide a guide for change. It is helpful to set a start date with the patient to begin implementing this program. It is also useful to review patient's goals. This demonstrates your interest and insures that the patient's goals are realistic and achievable.

Patients consistently report the benefits of the relaxation response technique, pacing activities, exercise, challenging negative self-talk, and diary keeping. If time is limited, focusing on these skills may be most productive. Otherwise, a chapter a week is a realistic pace to set.

With each week and each chapter, more observations and skills are added to the coping repertoire. Encourage patients to use and add to the skills—with the hope of achieving a synergism—not just to do them one at a time.

To encourage action, ask at follow-up visits what patients are learning from their diary keeping, relaxation response techniques, and activity pacing. Because the cognitive therapy skills can begin to challenge some basic assumptions and beliefs, patients may be reluctant to do the writing exercises. These are crucial to changing cognitive distortions and ineffective patterns of thinking. Encourage patients to bring these exercise sheets to their follow-up appointments or to keep a journal. Journaling can help patients become more comfortable with what goes on inside the mind and how it reacts to the world. Growing self-awareness can gently move patients into action. This movement toward maintenance of action over time is essential for behavioral change to occur and become a new standard of living.

The sequence of chapters in this workbook reflects the way the program is taught. The arrangement of topics is geared toward encouraging patient adherence to the program through the gradual build-up of pain management skills. Techniques that are easier to learn and provide more immediate results—such as relaxation response techniques and exercise—are presented first. Once patients have successfully adopted these skills into their lives, they receive positive inducement to continue with the more complex techniques—ones requiring long-term practice, introspection, and self-reflection— taught in later chapters.

Pain Flare-Up Management and Maintenance

Chapter 10 of the workbook addresses relapse prevention and pain flare-up management. Whichever technique the patient chooses to employ, either "coping with stages of pain" or the "panic plan," a copy of the plan should be kept in his or her record and periodically updated. Referral to the plan can then be made should he or she experience a pain flare-up. However, if the patient insists that a particular pain flare-up is different from what he or she usually experiences, a reassessment is necessary to rule out other developments. I have found that once patients become active participants in pain management through this program, they are the best judges of their own pain experience.

From here on, periodic inquiries about maintenance of skills such as relaxation response techniques (Chapter 3), mini-relaxations (Chapter 3), pacing activities (Chapter 4), strategies for response to negative emotional states (Chapters 5 and 6), reduced caffeine consumption (Chapter 7), and communication skills (Chapter 8) will also serve to reinforce behavioral change maintenance. If patients have stopped practicing these skills and are having increased difficulty with pain management, it may be necessary for you to identify the specific problems holding them back. For example, is the patient experiencing a setback because he or she was secretly hoping this program would cure his or her pain, and it didn't? Did he or she stop the program because it was going so well it didn't seem necessary anymore? Or is a separate life crisis distracting him or her from the pain management program? Once you have determined what issues are involved, you can set a date for the patient to get back into the program and then reinstitute a schedule of periodic checks on his or her skills practice.

A Final Note

I cannot emphasize enough what a rewarding experience it is to see people change, improve their quality of life, and feel more empowered in the face of some of the most difficult pain problems. Going to where the patient is in terms of his or her level of information, beliefs, and readiness to consider new directions in behavior and lifestyle practices is critical. Your important role in facilitating this process will have its own rewards.

Margaret A. Caudill, MD, PhD
Dartmouth Medical School
Manchester, NH

References

Paul Arnstein, Margaret Caudill, Carol Lynn Mandle, A. Norris, and Ralph Beasley, "Self-Efficacy as a Mediator of the Relationship Between Pain Intensity, Disability and Depression in Chronic Pain Patients," *Pain, 81*: 483–491, 1999.

Niels Becker, Per Sjogren, Per Bech, Alf Kornelius Olsen, and Jorgen Eriksen, "Treatment Outcome of Chronic Non-malignant Pain Patients Managed in a Danish Multidisciplinary Pain Centre Compared to General Practice: A Randomised Controlled Trial," *Pain, 84*: 203–211, 2000.

Nicola Biller, Paul Arnstein, Margaret Caudill, Carol Wells-Federman, and Carolyn Guberman, "Predicting Completion of a Cognitive-Behavioral Pain Management Program by Initial Measures of a Chronic Pain Patient's Readiness for Change. *Clinical Journal of Pain, 16*(4): 352–359, 2000.

Margaret Caudill, Richard Schnable, Patricia Zuttenneister, Herbert Benson, and Richard Friedman, "Decreased Clinic Use by Chronic Pain Patients: Response to Behavioral Medicine Intervention," *Clinical Journal of Pain, 7*: 305–310, 1991.

Thomas L. Delbanco, "Enriching the Doctor–Patient Relationship by Inviting the Patient's Perspective," *Annals of Internal Medicine, 116*: 414–418, 1992.

L. D. Egbert, G. E. Battit, C. E. Welch, and M. K. Bartlett, "Reduction of Post-operative Pain by Encouragement and Instruction of Patients: A Study of Doctor–Patient Rapport," *New England Journal of Medicine, 270*: 825–827, 1964.

Brent Q. Hafen, Kathryn J. Frandsen, Keith J. Karren, and Keith Hooker, *The Health Effects of Attitudes, Emotions and Relationships* (Provo, UT: EMS, 1992).

Judith K. Ockene, "Physician-Delivered Interventions for Smoking Cessation," *Preventive Medicine, 16*: 723–737, 1987.

Dennis Turk, Donald Meichenbaum, and Myles Genest, *Pain and Behavioral Medicine: A Cognitive-Behavioral Perspective* (New York: Guilford Press, 1985).

Perforated Worksheets and Other Materials

Pain Diary

Name _____

	Describe situation	Physical sensation (0–10)	Describe physical sensation	Emotional response (0–10)	Describe emotional response	Action taken, including medications
Monday Date:	⇒	⇒	⇒	⇒	⇒	⇒
Time 1:						
Time 2:						
Time 3:		Total:		Total:		
		Average:		Average:		
Tuesday Date:						
Time 1:						
Time 2:						
Time 3:		Total:		Total:		
		Average:		Average:		
Wednesday Date:						
Time 1:						
Time 2:						
Time 3:		Total:		Total:		
		Average:		Average:		

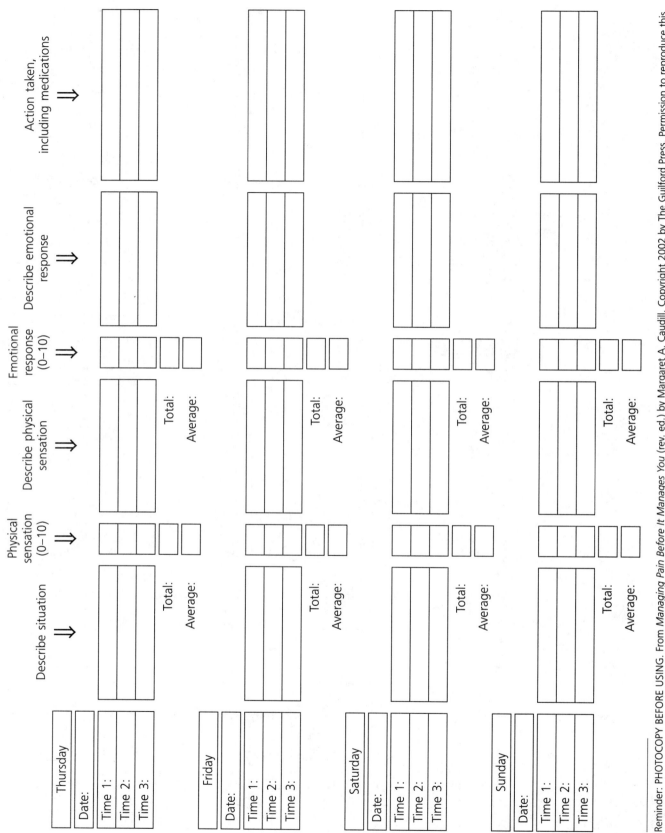

Relaxation Response Technique Diary

Complete the following weekly RR Diary. Next to each category indicate the appropriate information about your daily practice. Use this diary for the first three weeks to reinforce practice.

Date							
Time started							
Time stopped							
Place							
Position (e.g., lying down, sitting)							
Degree of relaxation at end (0–10) 0 = very relaxed 10 = very tense							
Effects on pain? Decrease = D Increase = I No change = NC							
Method (tape, exercise, visualization, other)							

Were there any problems that prevented you from practicing the RR daily? How can you solve the problem(s)? _____

_____

_____

_____

_____

_____

_____

_____

_____

Increasing Activities Worksheet

Date: _____ Name: _____

Make a list of activities that increase your pain and those that decrease your pain (refer to Chapter 4).

Activities that increase my pain	**Activities that decrease my pain**
Example: Washing dishes (standing)	Paying bills (sitting)

Can you *delegate* any of the activities associated with pain increases? (For example, bringing dirty laundry to the washing machine.) Star (*) the ones you can.

Delegate one activity this week. It will be _____

Choose one "increase pain" activity and time how long it takes to increase pain level by 2 points. Then choose a "decrease pain" activity from your list and time how long it takes for the pain to decrease again. Alternate between activities that increase and decrease your pain.

Example: Pain ↑ Activity = Wash dishes   Pain ↓ Activity = Pay bills

Wash dishes (10 mins.)	Sort bills from mail (15 mins.)
Wash dishes (10 mins.)	Write checks (15 mins.)
Wash dishes (10 mins.)	Address envelopes (10 mins.)

Activity that increases pain	**Activity that decreases pain**

Can you *adapt* any of the above activities so that they can be performed more easily? What would be some of the adaptations? (For example: sitting to fold laundry or peel vegetables; lying down to call a friend or listen to a book on tape; opening cabinet door under kitchen sink so that you can rest one foot on the shelf; putting bowls in sink to stir ingredients)

Food Diary Instructions

Time started: The time of day that you begin eating a meal.

Food/beverage: Record everything you eat and drink. Note such things as whether the food or beverage contained a sweetener substitute or whether it was a new product for you. Are you eating five servings of fruits and vegetables and six servings of grain products (including whole grains) per day?

Quantity: The amount that you ate or drank (1 cup, 8 oz. glass) or the plate portion (1/2, 1/4 of the dinner plate).

Time ended: The time at which you ended the meal you were recording. (If a number of your meals last 10 minutes or less, maybe you should consider eating more slowly.)

You may have to keep a food diary for many weeks before you see a relationship between foods and pain patterns.

Food Diary

Date: _____ Name: _____

Time started	Food/beverage	Quantity	Time ended

Daily Record of Automatic Thoughts (Self-Talk)

Date	Situation	Automatic thoughts	Physical response	Emotional response	Cognitive distortion	Changed thought

Weekly Feedback Sheet

Name: _____

Date: _____ Reporting for week of: _____

1. Record the daily averages of your physical sensation and emotional response below:

	Day 1	Day 2	Day 3	Day 4	Day 5	Day 6	Day 7	Weekly average
Physical sensation:	____	____	____	____	____	____	____	____
Emotional response:	____	____	____	____	____	____	____	____

If this is your first session, record your pain level now (on a scale of 0–10): ____

2. Over the past week, has your *physical sensation*:

Improved ____   Stayed the same ____   Become worse ____

Why do you think that your *physical sensation* has improved, stayed the same, or become worse?

_____

_____

Over the past week, has your *emotional response*:

Improved ____   Stayed the same ____   Become worse ____

Why do you think that your *emotional response* has improved, stayed the same, or become worse?

_____

_____

3. List all medication you are taking:

Name of medication	Dosage (mg)	Frequency*
_____	_____	_____
_____	_____	_____
_____	_____	_____
_____	_____	_____
_____	_____	_____
_____	_____	_____
_____	_____	_____

*How many times per day or per week do you take each medication?
If you take opioids, how many pills did you take for this week? ____

4. Did you receive any other pain treatments this week—for example, nerve blocks, physical therapy, acupuncture, etc.? _____

_____

_____

5. How many times this week did you do the following?

Relaxation response techniques _____   Mini-relaxations _____

6. For how long and how often did you do physical exercise this week?

Aerobic _____   Time _____   How often? _____

Stretching _____   Time _____   How often? _____

Strengthening _____   Time _____   How often? _____

7. What goal did you set for the week? _____
Did you accomplish it? (Y/N) _____   If you did not accomplish it, can you come up with a contingency plan that might help you succeed by identifying the obstacle and a solution to the obstacle?

Obstacle	Solution
_____	_____
_____	_____
_____	_____
_____	_____

8. Where did you find your pleasure this week? _____

_____

_____

9. Do you have any questions or problems? _____

_____

_____

10. To health care professionals: Is there any other information you wish to collect? Fill in before copying.

_____

_____

_____

_____

_____

_____

_____

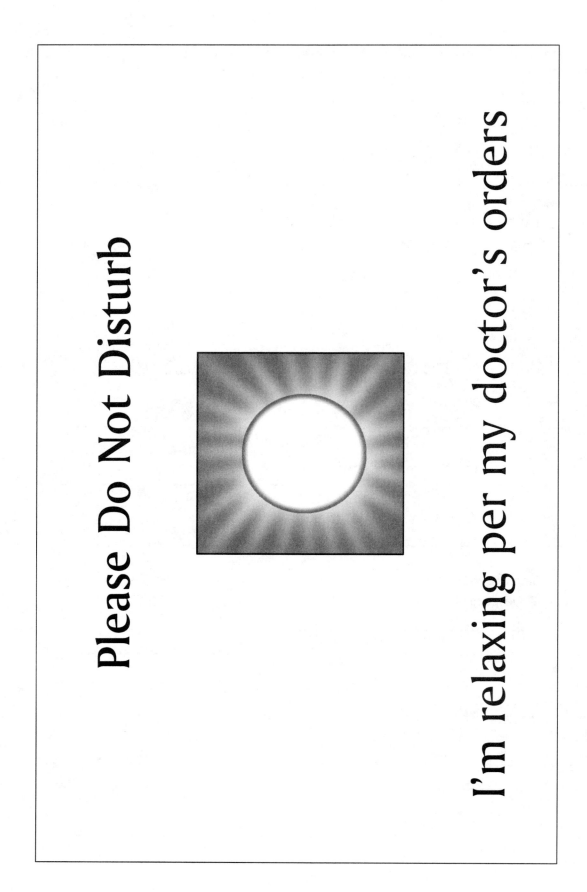

Letter to Health Care Professionals

Dear Health Care Professional:

Managing Pain Before It Manages You is a practical, patient-oriented workbook. It provides information on basic pain mechanisms, medical treatment of chronic pain, and multiple cognitive behavioral skills that can assist coping and functioning. This book can be used by patients alone but can be even more effective if supported by a health care professional who can guide the patient through the program and reinforce the book's information. The workbook was originally written to supplement a 10-visit group medical program for chronic pain management, but it can be used in individual therapy as well.

If you are a physician, nurse practitioner, or physician assistant, this book can supplement the pharmacological, interventional, and surgical treatments recommended to patients with chronic pain.

If you are a psychologist, social worker, or nurse, this workbook offers a complete, self-guided cognitive behavioral therapy program for your clients or patients. It may be used in patient education, in conjunction with other medical therapies, and in psychotherapy. Patients can use the workbook independently or as a formal 8- to 10-week individual or group program.

Efficacy of This Approach

Research has shown that health care professionals can play a critical role in facilitating a patient's response to therapeutic interventions, as well as in changing their behaviors (Egbert et al., 1964; Hafen et al., 1992; Ockene, 1987). For example, encouraging patients to discuss pain from their perspective and giving them information on self-management can increase patient adherence, reduce symptoms, and/or facilitate symptom management (Caudill et al., 1991; Delbanco, 1992). Applying a behavioral medicine model to symptom management acknowledges the complex biology, psychology, and sociology of an illness that needs to be considered in any therapeutic recommendation. The materials presented in this book are grounded in a behavioral medicine model, and they have been demonstrated to decrease symptoms and decrease clinic utilization by patients with chronic pain (Caudill et al., 1991; Becker et al., 2000). Furthermore, this intervention can increase self–efficacy, an important mediator of pain-related disability and depressive symptoms (Arnstein et al., 1999).

The Professional's Role in Facilitating This Program

> Those who do not feel pain, seldom think that it is felt.
> —*Samuel Johnson M.D., 1708–1784*

We can often best help patients with chronic pain by admitting the limits of our knowledge. There is much we don't know about chronic pain mechanisms for prevention or treatment. It is important to believe patients who report their pain experience. There is no objective measure of pain at this time. It is important for you and your patient to acknowledge that although living in pain is a challenge, there are many things that can be done to decrease symptoms and improve quality of life. If you do not feel comfortable evaluating and treating chronic pain, it is your obligation to refer the patient to someone who can.

Assessing and Encouraging Patient Readiness for Change

Teaching an appreciation of the biopsychosocial process from the time of the initial evaluation will lend validity to advising treatment that includes cognitive behavioral therapies. By exploring what other symptoms patients are experiencing in addition to their pain, the professional can help identify other stress-related symptoms, such as fatigue, memory problems, irritable bowel, muscle tension, shortness of breath, palpitations, irritability, and insomnia. Asking other specific questions in the psychosocial history can help get to other influencing issues and provide more mind–body connections for discussion; for example:

- "What functions or activities have been altered by your pain?" Humans are incredibly adaptable and are quite capable of using denial for coping. Detailing work inside and outside the home can give evidence for the magnitude of pain complaints.
- "From whom or what do you get your emotional or problem-solving support?" Behavioral medicine research has documented the positive power of support through close friends, spouses, and religious affiliation. However, many patients with chronic pain suffer isolation and despair.
- "In addition to your pain and dysfunction, what other stresses are you finding yourself having to cope with right now?" This can be a very revealing question. The losses incurred from unemployment or decreased work capacity alone can have economic, social, and self-esteem consequences of enormous importance.
- "Have you ever had a significant incident(s) of physical, emotional, or sexual abuse or trauma?" There is a very high positive response to this question in my practice. Such histories are important to uncover, as they influence how one might approach teaching the relaxation skills and may require individual treatment to put into perspective the differences between feeling vulnerable, not believed, and out of control after having been abused and when in chronic pain.
- "What do you think is going on? Do you have any fears or concerns about your pain?" The majority of patients have ideas (or fears) about the source or cause of their pain. For obvious reasons, addressing them may go along way in obtaining their willingness to see their part in pain management.
- "What do you want to get from your visit with me today?" This can be an important message to the patient that he or she has a right to have expectations regarding a visit and can be a good starting point in clarifying realistic expectations. This can be the perfect opening to discuss the roles of the health care professional and the patient toward reaching a common goal.

- "If I can't cure you today, what would be the next best thing?" This question stems from a common response of many patients to the last question. They will say, "You don't understand, doctor, I don't want my pain, so why would I want to manage it?" This again allows for the discussion of the nature of chronic pain and the reality of persistent pain. Early in treatment many people feel that acceptance of pain management is a condemnation to a life of pain even if a cure comes along, that somehow they will be excluded because they have accepted. This misunderstanding is important to clarify. Acceptance is dealing with the here and now; pain may be mandatory, but the suffering is definitely optional.

These questions can quickly give you an overview of the context of an individual's pain experience and lay the groundwork for establishing that pain is both stressful and affected by stress. It also sends the message that you are concerned about the pain and the person in pain. Listening to the responses of the patient to these questions helps set up realistic treatment expectations and orients treatment to the patient's level of understanding, in the context of his or her pain experience.

Patients in precontemplation (Biller et al., 2000) who have not thought about the relationship between behavior and pain can be asked just to read Chapters 1 through 5 of the workbook, without doing the exercises described. They can also begin keeping a pain diary, as described in Chapter 1, which will help them focus on just how their pain is affected by their daily activities and mood.

Patients are most ready to start *using* this workbook when they can acknowledge: (1) that changing their behavior may help them cope with or manage their pain, or (2) that they need new skills to handle the physical, emotional, and cognitive effects of pain on their lives.

Guiding Patients through the Workbook

When patients are ready for it, this workbook can provide a guide for change. It is helpful to set a start date with the patient to begin implementing this program. It is also useful to review patient's goals. This demonstrates your interest and insures that the patient's goals are realistic and achievable.

Patients consistently report the benefits of the relaxation response technique, pacing activities, exercise, challenging negative self-talk, and diary keeping. If time is limited, focusing on these skills may be most productive. Otherwise, a chapter a week is a realistic pace to set.

With each week and each chapter, more observations and skills are added to the coping repertoire. Encourage patients to use and add to the skills—with the hope of achieving a synergism—not just to do them one at a time.

To encourage action, ask at follow-up visits what patients are learning from their diary keeping, relaxation response techniques, and activity pacing. Because the cognitive therapy skills can begin to challenge some basic assumptions and beliefs, patients may be reluctant to do the writing exercises. These are crucial to changing cognitive distortions and ineffective patterns of thinking. Encourage patients to bring these exercise sheets to their follow-up appointments or to keep a journal. Journaling can help patients become more comfortable with what goes on inside the mind and how it reacts to the world. Growing self-awareness can gently move patients into action. This movement toward maintenance of action over time is essential for behavioral change to occur and become a new standard of living.

The sequence of chapters in this workbook reflects the way the program is taught. The arrangement of topics is geared toward encouraging patient adherence to the program through the gradual build-up of pain management skills. Techniques that are easier to learn and provide more immediate results—such as relaxation response techniques and exercise—are presented first. Once patients have successfully adopted these skills into their lives, they receive positive inducement to continue with the more complex techniques—ones requiring long-term practice, introspection, and self-reflection—taught in later chapters.

Pain Flare-Up Management and Maintenance

Chapter 10 of the workbook addresses relapse prevention and pain flare-up management. Whichever technique the patient chooses to employ, either "coping with stages of pain" or the "panic plan," a copy of the plan should be kept in his or her record and periodically updated. Referral to the plan can then be made should he or she experience a pain flare-up. However, if the patient insists that a particular pain flare-up is different from what he or she usually experiences, a reassessment is necessary to rule out other developments. I have found that once patients become active participants in pain management through this program, they are the best judges of their own pain experience.

From here on, periodic inquiries about maintenance of skills such as relaxation response techniques (Chapter 3), mini-relaxations (Chapter 3), pacing activities (Chapter 4), strategies for response to negative emotional states (Chapters 5 and 6), reduced caffeine consumption (Chapter 7), and communication skills (Chapter 8) will also serve to reinforce behavioral change maintenance. If patients have stopped practicing these skills and are having increased difficulty with pain management, it may be necessary for you to identify the specific problems holding them back. For example, is the patient experiencing a setback because he or she was secretly hoping this program would cure his or her pain, and it didn't? Did he or she stop the program because it was going so well it didn't seem necessary anymore? Or is a separate life crisis distracting him or her from the pain management program? Once you have determined what issues are involved, you can set a date for the patient to get back into the program and then reinstitute a schedule of periodic checks on his or her skills practice.

A Final Note

I cannot emphasize enough what a rewarding experience it is to see people change, improve their quality of life, and feel more empowered in the face of some of the most difficult pain problems. Going to where the patient is in terms of his or her level of information, beliefs, and readiness to consider new directions in behavior and lifestyle practices is critical. Your important role in facilitating this process will have its own rewards.

Margaret A. Caudill, MD, PhD
Dartmouth Medical School
Manchester, NH

References

Paul Arnstein, Margaret Caudill, Carol Lynn Mandle, A. Norris, and Ralph Beasley, "Self-Efficacy as a Mediator of the Relationship Between Pain Intensity, Disability and Depression in Chronic Pain Patients," *Pain, 81*: 483–491, 1999.

Niels Becker, Per Sjogren, Per Bech, Alf Kornelius Olsen, and Jorgen Eriksen, "Treatment Outcome of Chronic Non-malignant Pain Patients Managed in a Danish Multidisciplinary Pain Centre Compared to General Practice: A Randomised Controlled Trial," *Pain, 84*: 203–211, 2000.

Nicola Biller, Paul Arnstein, Margaret Caudill, Carol Wells-Federman, and Carolyn Guberman, "Predicting Completion of a Cognitive-Behavioral Pain Management Program by Initial Measures of a Chronic Pain Patient's Readiness for Change. *Clinical Journal of Pain, 16*(4): 352–359, 2000.

Margaret Caudill, Richard Schnable, Patricia Zuttenneister, Herbert Benson, and Richard Friedman, "Decreased Clinic Use by Chronic Pain Patients: Response to Behavioral Medicine Intervention," *Clinical Journal of Pain, 7*: 305–310, 1991.

Thomas L. Delbanco, "Enriching the Doctor–Patient Relationship by Inviting the Patient's Perspective," *Annals of Internal Medicine, 116*: 414–418, 1992.

L. D. Egbert, G. E. Battit, C. E. Welch, and M. K. Bartlett, "Reduction of Post-operative Pain by Encouragement and Instruction of Patients: A Study of Doctor–Patient Rapport," *New England Journal of Medicine, 270*: 825–827, 1964.

Brent Q. Hafen, Kathryn J. Frandsen, Keith J. Karren, and Keith Hooker, *The Health Effects of Attitudes, Emotions and Relationships* (Provo, UT: EMS, 1992).

Judith K. Ockene, "Physician-Delivered Interventions for Smoking Cessation," *Preventive Medicine, 16*: 723–737, 1987.

Dennis Turk, Donald Meichenbaum, and Myles Genest, *Pain and Behavioral Medicine: A Cognitive-Behavioral Perspective* (New York: Guilford Press, 1985).

To the Clinician:

Here are two convenient methods for ordering *Managing Pain Before It Manages You, Revised Edition*.

1. QUANTITY DISCOUNTS

For multiple copies of *Managing Pain Before It Manages You, Revised Edition*, see the discount schedule below. Simply multiply the discount price times the quantity you are ordering. Add 5% of your total order for shipping.

Quantity	List Price	Discount	Price per Book
1 book	$19.95	—	$19.95
2-9		10% off list price	$17.96
10+		15% off list price	$16.96

To order, please call toll-free 1-800-365-7006

2. CLIENT/PATIENT ORDER FORMS

Or, you may have your clients order directly from Guilford with the Client/Patient Order Form below. Client/Patient Order Forms are given priority attention. We also assure confidentiality. Customers using these order forms will be excluded from the Guilford mailing list and will receive no further correspondence. We suggest that you photocopy this order form for future use.

Priority Client / Patient Order Form

Send to:

GUILFORD PUBLICATIONS, INC.,
Dept. SELF, 72 Spring Street, New York, NY 10012

© CALL TOLL-FREE 1-800-365-7006
Mon.-Fri., 9am-5pm Eastern Time
(Be sure to tell the representative you are ordering from our priority client/patient order form.)
Or Call 212-431-9800
Fax 212-966-6708

Name

Address

City   State   Zip

Daytime Phone No. (   )

Method of Payment:

(All prices are in U.S. dollars. Payment must be made in U.S. dollars, payable on a U.S. bank)

☐ Check or Money Order Enclosed.

Bill my: ☐ MasterCard ☐ VISA ☐ American Express

Account No.   Exp. Date

☐☐☐☐ ☐☐☐☐ ☐☐☐☐ ☐☐☐☐ ☐☐ ☐☐

                              Month Year

Signature

(required for all credit card orders)

Name of recommending professional

Please Ship:

Qty.		Cat.#	Amount
1	**Managing Pain Before It Manages You, Revised Edition**	0718	**$19.95**
	Shipping (via Priority Mail - 1-2 week delivery)		**$4.50**
	In NY and PA, add sales tax / In Canada, add G.S.T.		
	Total		

For office use only

Priority Order

Note: Operator—set up as account type IT—Mail <u>No</u>—Rush Order
SHIP VIA FC